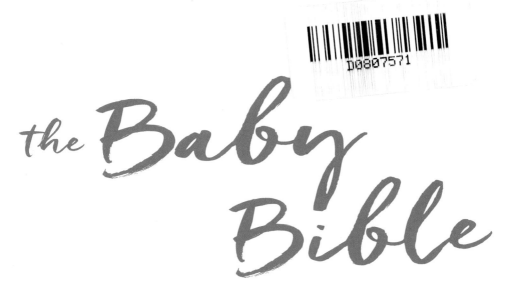

the Baby Bible

A guide to taking care of your bump, your baby and yourself

BEC JUDD

with LAUREN SAMS

ALLEN&UNWIN

Contents

The accidental mum   5
    The dream team   12

Before the bump   18
    Finding out I was going to be a mum   20

Month 1 (weeks 1–4)   26
    Being pregnant with Billie   28
    Interruption from an expert: Pregnancy 101   29
    The do's and don'ts   34
    Interruption from an expert: Nutrition during pregnancy   36
    Pregnancy exercise: The first trimester   40
    Interruption from an expert: Pelvic floor exercises   41
    Pregnancy skincare   43
    Interruption from an expert: Pregnancy and beauty products   49

Month 2 (weeks 5–8)   52
    Public or private?   54
    Interruption from an expert: What the hell is happening to my body?   57
    So . . . you're having more than one baby   61
    Interruption from an expert: Tests, tests, tests   64
    Interruption from an expert: Multiple pregnancy   67

Month 3 (weeks 9–13)   68
    How to style your bump   70
    Interruption from an expert: Genetic testing   74
    Finding out the sex   75
    Interruption from an expert: Twelve-week ultrasound (and other tests)   79

Month 4 (weeks 14–17)   84
    Dude, where's my abs?   86
    Interruption from an expert: All about diastasis recti   87
    Pregnancy exercise: The second trimester   90
    Interruption from an expert: Safe exercise during pregnancy   93
    Bec's workouts   98

Month 5 (weeks 18–21)   114
    Pregnancy hormones   116
    Birth classes: Yay or nay?   118
    Interruption from an expert: Second trimester ultrasound   120
    Eating for two . . . or three   123
    Gross things that are going to happen (sorry)   136

Month 6 (weeks 22–26)   138
    Baby gear: What do you really need?   140
    Styling the nursery   152

Month 7 (weeks 27–30)   160
  Babymoon time   162
  Interruption from an expert: Airline travel   167
  Pregnancy exercise: The third trimester   169
  Interruption from an expert: 28-week blood test   170
  Packing the baby bag   171
  Interruption from an expert: Third trimester ultrasound   177
  Birth plan   178

Month 8 (weeks 31–35)   180
  Giving birth to the twins   182
  The baby shower   183

Month 9 (weeks 36–40)   190
  Nesting—and relaxing   192
  Setting up your home   194

The big day   196
  Everything I know about labour   198
  Interruption from an expert: Everything Midwife Cath
    knows about labour   204

Your first few days as a mum   220
  Breastfeeding (or, how to use your boobs to keep your baby alive) 222
  Interruption from an expert: Everything you wanted to know
    about breastfeeding   225
  Conflicting advice   236
  Baby blues   238
  Not all postnatal depression looks the same   240

Recovery   244
  Your body after birth   246
  Interruption from an expert: Caring for your body post-birth   248

Home time   254
  Routines   256
  Interruption from an expert: Why you should wrap your baby   266
  Sleeping FAQs   268
  Interruption from an expert: Newborn routines   269
  Safe sleeping tips   283
  Baby gear: The stuff you'll need later   287
  Travel with a newborn   288
  Mum life hacks you never knew you needed   294

Final thoughts   296
Acknowledgements   299
Index   300

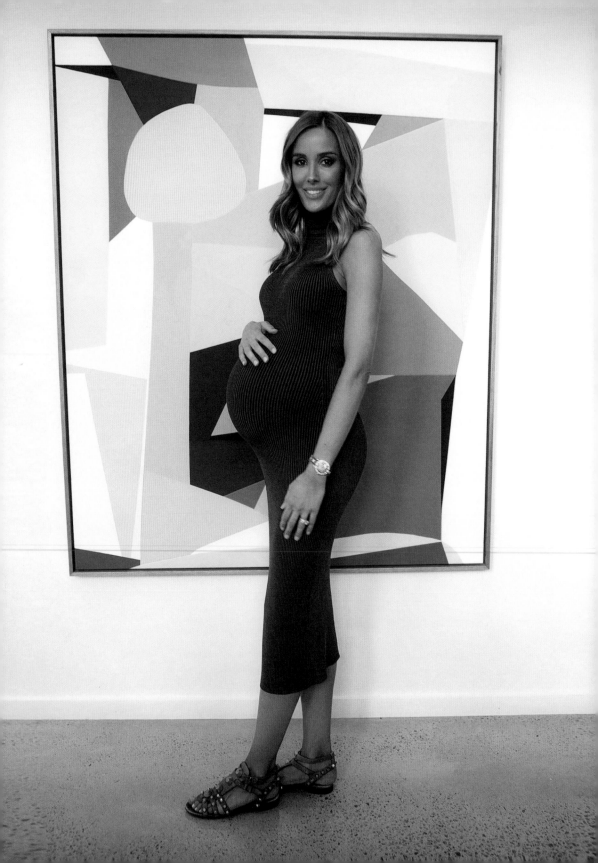

The accidental mum

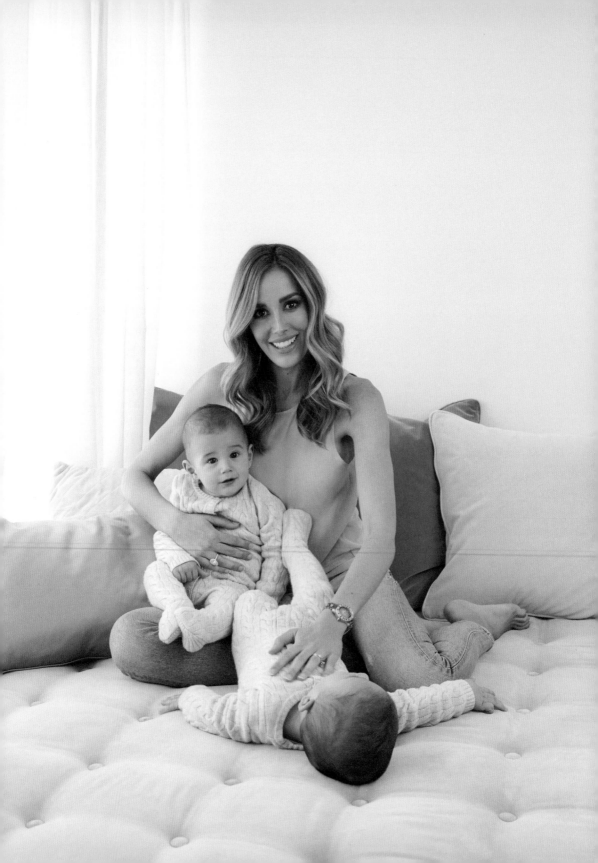

Hi, I'm Bec.

First up, congratulations! I hear you're having a baby. (Don't worry, nobody spilled—your skin looks amazing and you said no to sushi last night so I just had a hunch.)

Welcome to the Baby Roller-coaster. There are ups. There are downs. You'll probably throw up. You might lose the contents of your purse.

But hang in there.

You probably know by now that I have four kids. Four! I know. It's a lot. Four kids is new car territory. It's 'say goodbye to overseas holidays' land. (Four kids on a plane? I'd rather be on that plane with all the snakes, thanks very much.) It's a birthday party every weekend. It's a lot of sleepless nights.

It's full on.

But it's also the best thing I ever did.

The funny thing is, I can't quite believe I'm a mum of four. One? Sure. Two? No problem. But four kids? That's . . . a little much.

I often think of myself as an 'accidental mum' (not least because I did fall pregnant accidentally—more on that later) because I was never particularly maternal. You know that friend who is just desperate to have a baby? The one who can't walk past Cotton On Kids without having 'a little look'? The one who volunteers to hold the baby (literally anyone's baby), no matter where you are? The one who picked out their baby names before they even got their period?

Yeah, that was never me.

I love my kids, and I always wanted to have them someday, but people assume that because I have four kids, I must be all about kids. (I'll be honest: I'm not super into other kids. If my kids were the only kids I ever interacted with, that would be OK with me.) When I found out I was pregnant with Oscar, my eldest son, my first thought was: *Fuuuuuuuuuuuuuuuuuck.* Then: *I need a drink.* And then: *Fuuuuuuuuuuuuuuuuuuck.*

When I had Oscar, I honestly felt like I had ruined my life. What had I been thinking, having a child? Babies were so needy. So loud. So oblivious to the fact that their parents need sleep. I felt like Oscar was this little alien, invading our house and our lives. I had no idea how to speak his language, how to negotiate with him. I felt lost and out of control.

And then I got help. And then—almost overnight—everything changed.

And that, of course, is what you're here for: help. Whether you're a first-time mum or this isn't your first baby rodeo (sidenote: how cute would baby cowboy boots be?), I am here for you. Because as much as I've been an accidental mum of sorts, I've also been lucky enough to surround myself with some of the most brilliant pregnancy and baby experts in Australia, and from them I've learned so much. Now it's time for me to pass on what I've learned from three pregnancies and four children to you.

Over the last six years—and especially with the recent addition of my twins, Tom and Darcy—I've had so many people ask me: 'How do you do it?' My answer is probably the same as anyone else's: I'm not really sure, but I do. Sometimes I still feel like I'm flying by the seat of my pants . . . but other days, I feel like I've got a handle on things. I will always champion love, warmth, good food, routine, asking for help and not being too hard on yourself. (And let's get that mother guilt thing out of the way early: the fact you may even worry that you are not a good enough mother proves that you already are. End of story.)

This book will share with you how I did it: three pregnancies and deliveries and four gorgeous newborn babies. From carrying your baby, delivering it, feeding it and raising it, there are so many ways in which us mums can do things. If the way you mother is done safely, with love, and you and your child are happy, then it is perfect—don't let anybody tell you it's not.

Believe me, I've been through it all. From bottle-fed babies to a perfect breastfeeder, from a natural vaginal delivery to an emergency caesarean, from breastfeeding my first baby through the rungs in his cot to get him to sleep, to faultless routine babies who slept all night from six weeks of age, I have experienced almost everything that motherhood could throw at me.

I'm not an expert, but over the past six years, I've learned a lot. And now I want to share what I've learned—as well as some of the genius advice and knowledge from my dream team (more on them later)—with you. Because having a baby is amazing, but it can also be scary and overwhelming. There's so much advice out there, it's hard to know what to follow. Here's what you can expect from this book: no BS, just the truth. I'm so excited to share this beautiful time with you. Let's get going, shall we?

How to use this book

While the chapters are laid out chronologically (from month 1 to having a newborn), you can pick up chapters at random to figure out what's going on with your changing body, mind and mood at that very moment.

The book is mainly based on my experiences, but whenever I have included expert knowledge from my dream team, you'll see the heading 'Interruption from an expert'. And while every effort has been made to include the most current and accurate information, what we know about pregnancy and birth can change, so please ask your doctor if you're unsure about anything.

A little note, before we begin

One thing this book will never do is judge other mums. Judging other women's bodies, boobs and baby-rearing skills seems to be a national sport these days, but you will *not* find that kind of stuff here. Look, we all do things differently and that is fine. There will be no judgement about breastfeeding or bottle-feeding, co-sleeping or strict baby routines, or mums who want to have a little wedge of brie when seven months pregnant. And I'd encourage you to do the same: after all, mums have enough to deal with every single day without worrying what everyone else is thinking of their parenting skills. Let's all agree, before we get going, that as long as our babies are safe and loved, they will be OK.

I know it's a cliché, but we ladies need to support one another. Growing a baby and being a mother is such a privilege—but it's also tricky, trying and exhausting. Be kind to one another and know that we all have different ideas. That's OK. Being awful to one another isn't.

Good luck—and try not to chuck.

The moment I knew I *would* have kids

OK, so I know I told you I was never the most maternal person . . . but when I met Chris, my husband, I knew I wanted to have kids with him. Anyone else know that feeling? Before I met Chris, I'd never been in love before—actually, I'd never even had a proper boyfriend. When we met (at a Perth pub after waaaaay too many Bacardi Breezers), I was immediately infatuated. Like in one of those cartoons where the light bulb appears over your head. It was just like 'Ding ding ding, here he is'.

Unfortunately, I was due to go overseas for a modelling job pretty much as soon as I met him, and Chris . . . well, Chris still had a girlfriend. But a few months later, when I got back, Chris had broken up with his girlfriend and we were ready to give it a crack. It was full on, right from the beginning: just complete love. I'd never felt anything like it before, and I knew that it was real.

A month or so in, I vividly remember standing in his kitchen, doing the dishes together, and Chris said, 'What do you reckon about us? Do you think we'll stay together forever?' I was trying my best to be casual (but inside I was screaming, 'YES YES YES YES') and said something smooth like, 'Oh, yeah.' And then Chris said, 'How many kids do you think we should have?' And that was it: kids. Another light bulb went off and I knew that my life was about to change. And oh boy, did it ever!

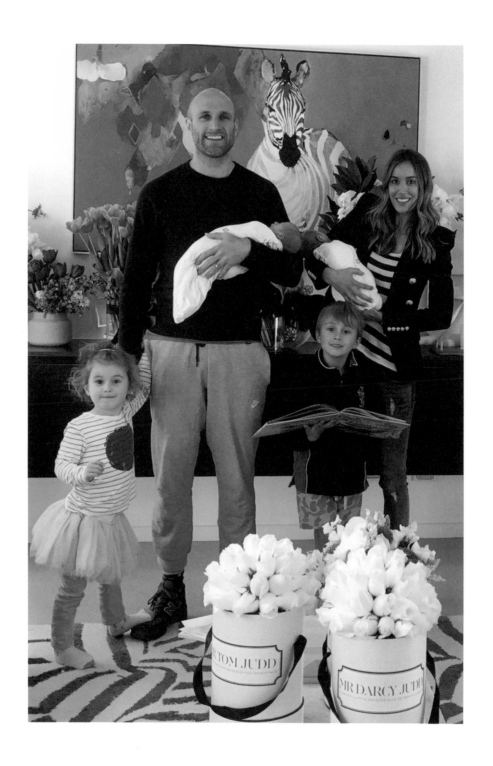

The dream team

Before we start, I want to introduce you to my personal pregnancy, baby and birth dream team. Without these men and women—and my husband, of course—I wouldn't have my four beautiful kids. I owe them so much for their smarts, expertise, care and understanding. They're all experts in their fields, and they have so much knowledge to share with you. I'm proud to call them my friends, and I'm so happy they're sharing their wisdom with you in this book. Here's a little about each of them.

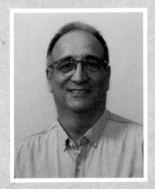

The Obstetrician
Dr Len Kliman
OAM, MBBS, FRANZCOG

Dr Len Kliman is an obstetrician and gynaecologist practising in Melbourne. In his 40-plus-year career, he has delivered more than 20,000 babies. Graduating from the University of Melbourne in 1977, Dr Kliman was a resident medical officer at the Royal Melbourne Hospital for two years. He completed his obstetrics and gynaecology training at the Royal Women's Hospital, where he was a consultant obstetrician and gynaecologist from 1986 to 2000. He has also practised obstetrics and gynaecology in the UK and the USA, where he specialised in high-risk pregnancies and chemical dependency.

Since 2002 Dr Kliman has been the Chairman of Obstetrics at the Epworth Freemasons Hospital in Melbourne, where he also continues to teach medical students, midwives and obstetric and gynaecological trainees for the Royal Australian and New Zealand College of Obstetricians and Gynaecologists. Dr Kliman is one of Melbourne's most experienced obstetricians and gynaecologists, having supervised the care of thousands of public and private patients.

In 2017 Dr Kliman received a Medal of the Order of Australia for outstanding service to medicine in the field of obstetrics and gynaecology.

Dr Kliman is married with two children. He loves his Vespa, scuba diving and, of course, babies. He is also a Collingwood fan, something I try not to hold against him.

See drlenkliman.com.au.

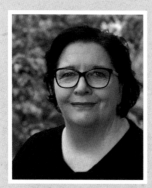

The Midwife
Cathryn Curtin
RN, RM, MCH
. . . .

Cath Curtin—or as I know her, Midwife Cath—is a trusted expert in women's health, pre-pregnancy, antenatal care and education, pregnancy, labour and birth, postnatal care, breastfeeding and parenting. In her 42-year career, she has delivered more than 10,000 babies.

Trained and fully qualified as a nurse, midwife, and maternal and child health nurse, Cath has an incomparable depth of experience. Thousands of parents have attended her monthly master classes on childbirth education, and sleep and settling.

Cath has a private consulting business, allowing her to work directly with parents over the phone or via FaceTime or Skype. These sessions focus on problem-solving specific challenges such as sleeping and feeding, as well as general parenting issues for newborn babies to toddlers. She also consults on issues concerning the health of the mother, especially anxiety and postnatal depression. Cath works with parents across Australia and internationally.

Her book, *The First Six Weeks*, was published by Allen & Unwin in 2016, and is now being translated for international markets. For more, head to **midwifecath.com.au**.

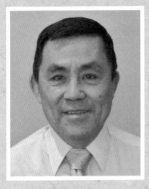

The Ultrasound Expert
Dr Andrew C.C. Ngu
MBBS, FRANZCOG, DDU, COGU
. . . .

Dr Andrew Ngu has been in practice performing in obstetrics and gynaecology ultrasound since 1984 and is one of the pioneers in this field. He graduated in medicine at Monash University, Melbourne, in 1976 and obtained his specialist degree in obstetrics and gynaecology in 1986. He worked at the ultrasound department at Royal Women's Hospital, Melbourne, from 1986 till 2010, and has been the deputy director and relieving director of the department.

Not only did Dr Ngu practise at the ultrasound department at the Royal Women's Hospital for almost 25 years, he was also incredibly active in setting standards in obstetrics and gynaecology ultrasound globally. As a result, he was elected to the board of the International Society of Ultrasound in Obstetrics and Gynaecology (ISUOG) in 2004, and was the second representative on that board outside of Europe and the USA. He served as the president of ISUOG from 2014 to 2016.

Dr Ngu also served on the Australasian Society for Ultrasound Medicine (ASUM), and was president from 1998 to 2000. During his presidency at ASUM he set up the first Ultrasound School in Kuala Lumpur, Malaysia, to teach ultrasound in his home country. To date, the school has had over 150 graduates. He is also a founding director of the Australian Institute of Healthcare Education (AIHE) in Sydney where ultrasound degrees are offered.

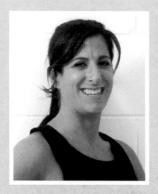

The Women's Health Physiotherapist
Shira Kramer
BPhty (Hons), PGCertPhysio (Exercise for Women)

Shira Kramer is one of Australia's leading women's health and fitness professionals. She is an experienced physiotherapist, fitness leader, international presenter and the founder of BeActive Physio in Melbourne. Shira is also a mother to two beautiful boys.

As well as her professional expertise, Shira understands the demands of motherhood, and has considered this when developing her program, 'Restore Your Core'. Revolutionary and the first of its kind, Shira's online exercise program is designed to help women return to exercise safely in the postpartum period. You can start restoring your own core on her website, **shirakramer.com.au**.

A passionate advocate for women's health, Shira is a proud ambassador for the Pelvic Floor First campaign. Shira believes all women deserve to be trained safely and effectively, especially through pregnancy, postpartum and all the stages that follow. She delivers education programs to both physiotherapists and fitness professionals on a regular basis, presenting at conferences and in university settings. A renowned global speaker and mentor for women's health and wellness, Shira's passion is to keep women active from all ages and stages in life.

My pelvic floor totally owes her a beer.

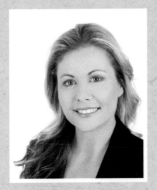

The Paediatric Sleep Expert

Amanda McGill

BMid, GradCertPaedSleepSci

. . . .

Amanda McGill is a highly esteemed Australian paediatric sleep specialist and postnatal midwife.

Dedicated to helping families thrive, Amanda has a graduate certificate in paediatric sleep science and a bachelor's degree in midwifery science. She also has qualifications in early childhood education and care, maternity and social science (psychology).

Amanda has been bringing harmony to families for over seventeen years by putting infant and child sleep issues to rest. Her passion and work have taken her all over the world.

Amanda is the co-founder of the Australian Nanny Association (ANA), and also the owner and operator of Nest Nannies, a postnatal maternity and night nanny agency located in Melbourne. Her website is **amandamcgill.com.au** and the Nest Nannies website is **nestnannies.com.au**.

Amanda helped me get my babies to sleep well—if I owe Shira a beer, I owe Amanda the whole damn case.

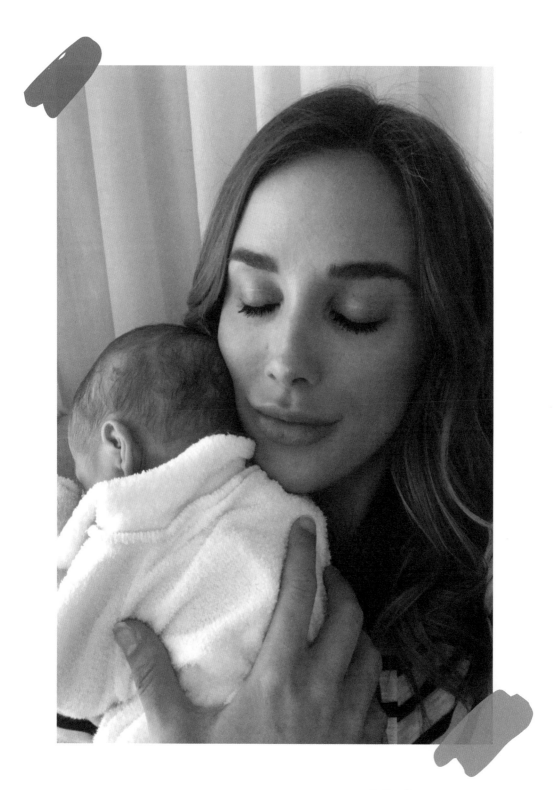

We've already established I wasn't exactly lining up to be a mum . . . but at the same time, I always knew kids were in my future. I was lucky enough to fall pregnant relatively easily with all three pregnancies (and as you'll find out shortly, a little *too* easily with one in particular). Without sounding too much like a *Law and Order* episode (dun, dun), these are their stories.

Before the bump

Finding out I was going to be a mum

I found out I was pregnant with Oscar the day before my hen's party.

I know.

What a bummer, right?

I actually couldn't believe it. Chris and I thought we were being careful by not having sex on days I was ovulating. Little did I know, I was not actually ovulating when I thought I was. I was dropping eggs left, right and centre— and I had no idea. Let this be a lesson to you!

So there I was, getting ready for my hen's do, when a pregnancy test (from a scare about two years earlier) fell out of a cupboard I was fishing around in. On a whim, I decided to do it. I'd had a bit of weird cramping going on, which was strange as I wasn't due for my period for a few days, and it *never* came early. Like, not once in my life had it come early. My reproductive cycle is the definition of clockwork. So when the pregnancy test literally fell in my lap it was like there was this little voice in my head saying, 'Do it. Piss on that stick. You must.' And so I did.

And then I saw those two little lines show up. I couldn't believe it: I was meant to be slamming tequila shots the next day. I went to the chemist and bought about six more tests (just to be certain, you know) and sure enough, one by one, they showed up positive. Positive, positive, positive.

Oh shit. We were going to have a baby.

The next day, I nursed a single glass of champagne (my doctor said it was OK; I hung up before he could change his mind). When I told my girlfriends that I was pregnant, they were . . . well, a little sad, to be honest! Their faces dropped when I told them the news. I could tell they were thinking, *But what about the hen's? What about the wedding? What about this entire summer?* It was like I'd been stolen from them—by a foetus, no less—without any warning. A part of me felt the same way. I was usually the ringleader, but now I was sitting in the corner at my own hen's party, still in shock that I, of all people—the least maternal one—was pregnant.

While I was happy to be pregnant, I was also quite overwhelmed. I was the first one in my friendship group to fall pregnant, and that was daunting. I knew we'd start trying for children sometime after we got married, but that was at least twelve months away. This was not part of the plan! And for someone like me—a hardcore, type-A planner—this was not good. I like to feel prepared, and falling pregnant accidentally doesn't exactly make you feel like you've got your shit together. Besides all that, Chris and I wanted to enjoy married life first. (Sidenote: what does that even mean? People say it all the time and I still don't really know what it's about.) We lived a pretty self-absorbed lifestyle in Prahran—shopping, eating, heading out to bars and clubs. How the hell would a baby fit into that lifestyle?!

Chris and I got married on New Year's Eve, 2010, and by then, I was ten weeks pregnant. Again, I babysat one glass of bubbles, and watched as our families and friends flocked to the fancypants cocktail bar we'd basically mortgaged our house to be able to afford. By that stage, we'd told our families, and my best girlfriends knew, but nobody else at the wedding did. Once more, I felt like I'd been ripped off on the biggest night of my life (at that point). Anybody who knows me in real life (or on Instagram!) knows that I love a boogie and a cocktail (or five). Everyone was having a ball; people kept running over and telling me, 'This is the best wedding EVERRRRRRRRRRRRR.' While I was ecstatic that everyone was enjoying the night so much, I couldn't help but wish I could experience it like they were. I was exhausted and sore and asked Chris if we could go home at 11 p.m.—despite having booked the venue till 2 a.m. (and with the NYE fireworks display still to come). I was buggered and flat and honestly, a little envious of everyone else. Chris was in shock. 'You can't bloody leave your own wedding early!' he said. He was right, but I was wrecked. We compromised and I went and sat in the bridal 'green room' for half an hour with my girlfriends. They were all giggly and drunk and having a ball. They pepped me up with a laugh, handed me a strong coffee and helped me cheer up. Thank god for girlfriends, hey? I got my second wind and ended up carving up the dance floor until 3 a.m.

After the wedding, I started to get pretty excited about being pregnant, and let go of some of the feelings that were holding me back. I mean, oh my god! I got pregnant without even trying to. In fact, I got pregnant while actively trying *not* to. Thinking this way really shifted my mindset and made me feel very lucky. After that, I really started to embrace this new chapter of my life. I felt proud and happy and ready. I was pregnant. It had taken some

How to know when you're ovulating

OK, so if you're pregnant, you probably already have an idea of when you ovulated (or maybe you were like me and had no idea. Surprise!). First up, ovulation is when you release an egg, ready to meet up with some sperm. There are a few ways to figure out when you're likely to ovulate.

Calendar method: If you have a regular cycle (i.e. it's the same number of days every month), count back fourteen days from when you're expecting your next period. Your fertile window (i.e. when you should be Doing It) is this day, and the five days before it. This is an easy method, but it's not super accurate (cases in point: Oscar and Billie Judd).

Ovulation predictor kits: You can buy kits (a little bit like home pregnancy tests) that will help determine when you're likely to be ovulating. There are two types of kits—one tests your urine, one looks at your saliva. You test every day, and they'll show a positive result on the days you're ovulating.

Analysing ovulation symptoms: Lots of women swear by tracking their basal body temperature (BBT) and cervical mucus for a few cycles to try to determine when they ovulate. You can get apps to help you do this, but you'll also need a special thermometer to record your BBT (your lowest body temperature in a 24-hour period). On the day after you ovulate, you should see an increase in this, of 0.5 to 1 degree Celsius. This temperature increase typically lasts until your next period. With cervical mucus, you'll notice an increase in the amount and a change in texture when you're ovulating.

getting used to, but it was real. I was a real pregnant person. How cool is that?

Looking back, my pregnancy with Oscar was so easy. Soon I actually found that I loved being pregnant. I had a few symptoms—nosebleeds (weird, right? I'd be walking down the street and—psshh! My nose would bleed like a goddamn tap), sore boobs, fatigue and minor cramping of my uterus (which is common in early pregnancy), but mostly, it was such a dream. The one thing that totally took me by surprise was the hunger. Hunger like you have never, ever experienced before. Hunger that makes you pull into the nearest drive-through and order everything off the menu. Hunger that takes over your mind and will not allow you to think of anything else until you've quietened the rumble in your tummy. Hunger that is like, 'Feed me now, Bec, or I will really mess you up.' One day, I was so hungry I could barely stand. There was nothing in the fridge, and only a jar of bicarb soda in the pantry. I almost cried. Then I remembered there was a stale piece of bread in the freezer . . . it looked mangled and gross, but I chucked it in the toaster, slathered some butter on it, and honestly, it was one of the best things I've ever eaten.

Being pregnant with Oscar was the most wonderful adventure. I can vividly recall the first time I saw his little heartbeat on the ultrasound, and the first time I felt him move inside me. It is truly other-worldly to feel a real person move inside you, it really is. It's a very visceral reminder that you're actually carrying a life inside you. A new life. There aren't really words to describe it, but it made me feel lucky to be a woman and be able to experience this miracle. I was so excited every single day of my pregnancy. It's not often that, as an adult, you get to do something for the first time, but being pregnant for the first time is a new surprise and adventure every single day.

And then there was Billie

Because I'd fallen pregnant so easily with Oscar (read: got knocked up totally by accident), I assumed getting pregnant a second time would be a breeze. You know, the old story: when a man and a woman love each other very much, and the man does all the washing up for a while . . . babies are made. Chris and I had decided to go for number two when Oscar was eighteen months old.

By then, he was such a chatty, fun little person. We were all having a ball and thought, why not do this again? The initial difficulties had all been forgotten— Oscar slept well, ate like a mini Carlton player and was generally a happy little Vegemite.

So we started trying for our second baby. Because Oscar had come along without us trying at all, we figured that falling pregnant again would be just as simple.

We started tracking my ovulation cycles and dutifully having sex on day 14, which is when your eggs are down to party with some sperm. The first month, nothing happened.

OK, we thought. It's only one month. Gotta keep trying.

The second month, nothing happened.

OK.

The third month, Chris was away playing footy. I briefly contemplated getting him to leave me a little sample jar before thinking better of it and getting a good night's sleep, instead.

The fourth month, I was away filming. Bloody hell, I thought. Is this ever going to happen?

I'm a bit of a control freak, and the idea of not being able to control my fertility was starting to make me anxious. So I booked an appointment with an acupuncturist who specialised in ovulation. I was all ready to go, when I noticed my boobs were a little sore. I took a pregnancy test that morning, expecting a negative as I'd been away on Hamilton Island when I was ovulating and—whaddya know?—I was pregnant. Hello, Billie Judd!

It turned out that I had no idea when I was actually ovulating. I assumed that—like most women—I ovulated around day 14, but that wasn't the case for me. I was ovulating around day 11, and so Chris and I were completely missing our window to get me pregnant. Luckily, in that fourth month, we'd had sex literally just before I went to the airport . . . which just happened to be day 11. Phew!

I called the acupuncturist and told her I didn't need to come in after all. And then I did a crazy happy dance—I was going to be a mum again, and it was so bloody exciting.

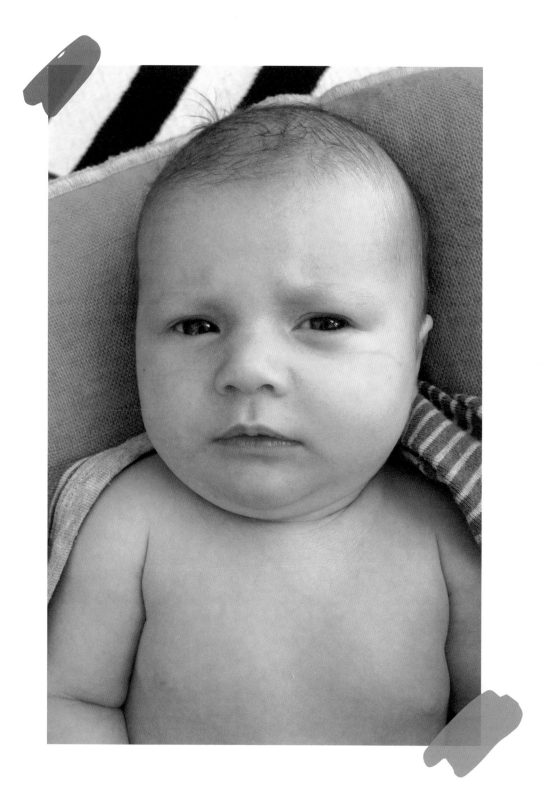

weeks 1–4

What's happening with baby

Yay! You're pregnant.

Well. Almost.

For the first two weeks of this month, you're actually not really pregnant—your body is preparing for ovulation like normal. When egg meets sperm, though—about three weeks after the first day of your last period—you'll be officially knocked up.

That fertilised egg will move down the Fallopian tubes to the uterus, and wedge itself nicely in the lining. Once this happens, your little egg becomes an embryo.

What's happening with you

Not much, to be honest. The pregnancy hormone, human chorionic gonadotropin (or hCG), is starting to rise. When you take a pregnancy test next month, it'll be positive due to the presence of that hormone.

Size-wise . . .

We're talking poppyseeds. I know, tiny, right? Biology is mind-blowing.

Month 1

Being pregnant with Billie

Being pregnant with Billie was a hugely different experience from my first time round. Chris and I were building a house, my career had really taken off, and of course, we had Oscar to consider and take care of. I didn't have time to worry about the things I worried about with Oscar. When you're first pregnant, you track every milestone and obsess over every symptom. With Billie, I barely knew what week I was up to.

As with Oscar, my pregnancy with Billie was pretty easy. I had nosebleeds again, and I was tired at first, but apart from that, I was lucky to feel well throughout the nine months.

At the end, I had a lot of pelvic pain because Billie's head was so far down. Every time I coughed or sneezed, I pissed my pants. So that wasn't a lot of fun. Unfortunately for me, Billie was quite content to rest her little head just on top of my cervix . . . for, like, three months. All my pelvic floor work is because of her.

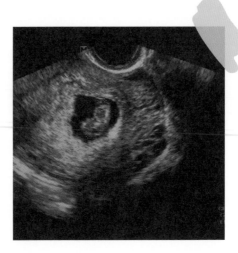

I see you, Billie!

Interruption from an expert

Pregnancy 101

OK, I know you have questions—yep, even the one about doing it when you're up the duff. It can be kind of confusing to keep track of everything that's meant to be bad for you and your baby—and even harder to figure out exactly *why* this stuff should be avoided. So I asked my obstetrician, Dr Len Kliman, to break it all down for us. Thanks, Dr Len.

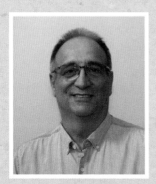

The Obstetrician

Dr Len Kliman

Can I still eat fish?

Yes. Fish is an excellent source of omega-3 fatty acids, which are vital to healthy brain development. There have been numerous studies showing that mothers who eat fish regularly during pregnancy have babies with improved neurodevelopment.

However, all fish contains mercury, and mercury consumption is associated with foetal brain damage if eaten in large quantities. To minimise your risk, avoid eating flake, swordfish, orange roughy and tuna (both tinned and fresh). Keep anchovies, herring, sardines, mackerel, salmon, trout and whiting on the menu—they're great sources of omega-3 fatty acids and have low levels of mercury.

If you can't eat fish, be sure to supplement your diet with an omega-3 fatty acid vitamin.

Can I drink?

I know you'd love me to say yes but ... the answer is no, not safely. While there have been a few interesting studies that show that one or two drinks per week is safe for the foetus, these studies were quite small and can't be considered definitive. Drinking poses big risks to the foetus, like growth restriction, foetal alcohol syndrome (a group of abnormalities associated with high alcohol intake or binge drinking) and delayed intellectual and social development in the first few years of life. The safest thing to do is not drink at all. Save up that champagne for when you see your baby for the first time!

Pleeeeease tell me I can still drink coffee.

Pregnant women are told to avoid too much caffeine mainly because there's no good scientific data that shows its effects during pregnancy. Despite this, it's believed that caffeine, especially in moderate amounts, poses very little risk of decreased foetal growth or abnormalities, or increased risk of miscarriage. But to be safe, limit your consumption of caffeine in all its forms—coffee, tea, chocolate, soft drinks—to 300 milligrams a day. Luckily, 300 milligrams is still quite a bit—so yes, you can absolutely have your coffee, and drink it, too. This is a rough guide so you can estimate your intake:

* 30 millilitre espresso = 60 milligrams caffeine
* cup of tea = 50 milligrams caffeine
* can of Coke or Diet Coke = 45 milligrams caffeine.

Can I have sex?

I am invariably asked about this by a tentative male partner at the first visit.

The short answer is, yes. There's no problem having sexual intercourse in a normal pregnancy. In theory, there is the risk of premature labour due to prostaglandins in semen and the release of the hormone oxytocin associated with orgasm (both of which have been shown to stimulate labour). However, numerous studies have shown that there is no increased risk of premature delivery related to intercourse and the release of these substances is of theoretical risk only and should not be of any concern.

In saying that, if you have obstetric complications you should always ask your obstetrician if it is safe to have intercourse in pregnancy. We're talking things like vaginal bleeding, placenta praevia, a cervical suture or if you've been told you're at risk of premature delivery.

I get crazy hay fever. Can I take antihistamines?

Yes. In fact, many pregnant women take antihistamines during pregnancy even if they're not prone to hay fever, as antihistamines have an anti-nauseant action, making them great for treating morning sickness.

There are two types of antihistamines: first generation and second generation.

First generation antihistamines (like Polaramine) are absolutely safe to use at any time during pregnancy. They can help alleviate morning sickness and relieve hay fever and allergy problems. You may, however, experience some drowsiness.

Second generation antihistamines (like Claratyne) are safe to use after twelve weeks' gestation. These aren't very useful in alleviating nausea, but they're great for combating hay fever and allergy problems.

What about Panadol? Nurofen? Other stuff like that?

Most over-the-counter medications are perfectly safe to use during pregnancy. Nurofen and other anti-inflammatories are not recommended after 24 weeks as they can affect the foetal heart, but Panadol and other paracetamol products are fine, as are nasal sprays and most cough mixtures and throat lozenges. If in doubt, ring your doctor or local medical hotline.

I've got a cat. Is that OK?

There's a small risk of contracting toxoplasmosis—a parasitic infection found in cat faeces—when pregnant, but in Australia our rates are very, very low. You can absolutely keep your cat, but take the following precautions:

* Don't feed your cat raw meat (another source of the infection).
* Have someone else clean the cat's litter tray.
* Wear gloves when gardening, in case your cat has soiled in the garden.
* Cook meat thoroughly, especially beef and pork (again, a potential source of the infection).

Can I work out?

Yes, absolutely. Cardio exercise and core strength workouts have a number of positive benefits for pregnant women, ranging from the physical to the psychological. Regular exercise has been linked to a reduction in the risk of pre-eclampsia, gestational diabetes and even your chances of having a caesarean section. Safe exercises include walking, jogging, low-impact aerobics, Pilates, yoga and swimming. You could also look for specialist prenatal exercise classes for pregnant women.

Always check with your doctor before starting a new exercise program when pregnant, particularly if you are either underweight or overweight, are a smoker, or have one of the following conditions:

* anaemia
* unevaluated maternal cardiac arrhythmia
* chronic bronchitis
* type 1 diabetes
* extreme intra-uterine growth restriction
* orthopaedic limitations.

There are some risks involved in exercising during pregnancy, but by following the guidelines above, you'll be able to avoid them. Extreme physical activity raises your core temperature to a level that may be harmful to your baby, but going for a half-hour jog or doing a yoga class three times a week will not pose a risk.

There are a few women who should not exercise during pregnancy, though. If you have any of the following conditions, please avoid exercising without consulting your obstetrician:
* significant heart disease
* significant lung disease
* incompetent cervix or cervical suture
* multiple gestation with the risk of premature labour
* persistent second or third trimester bleeding
* placenta praevia after 26 weeks
* ruptured membranes
* any risk of premature labour
* pre-eclampsia or pregnancy-induced hypertension
* severe anaemia.

Can I go in a spa bath?

When your temperature is raised during pregnancy, there's an increased risk of foetal abnormalities like spina bifida. While a bath at home in your bathroom is unlikely to raise your body temperature above 39 degrees Celsius (the point at which abnormalities can occur), spa baths are designed to reach 40 degrees, so may pose a risk. If you are visiting a spa, limit your time in the tub to ten minutes or less. Get out if you feel unwell or start to sweat excessively. And if you are worried, take your temperature while you're in the bath or spa—and, of course, if your temp rises above 39 degrees, hop out!

The do's and don'ts

You've probably heard rumours that pregnant women basically can't do anything. No wine, no soft cheese, no monster truck rallies—no fun stuff, right? While it's true we need to avoid delicious things like runny camembert and swirls of soft serve for the next nine or so months, there are also issues like food safety to consider.

Foods to avoid

Let's get to the important stuff first: food. Everyone knows pregnant women aren't meant to have soft cheese or sashimi . . . but why? Because they pose the risk of carrying the bacterial infection listeria, which—although very uncommon—can lead to miscarriage if not treated. Listeria is a bit like the flu—you get chills, fever, aches and pains, and diarrhoea. Strangely enough, listeria can often present up to *three weeks* after you eat the contaminated food.

The list of foods commonly associated with listeria—and therefore, which you need to avoid—are:
* unpasteurised milk products
* soft cheeses, including ricotta and feta
* raw seafood
* unwashed fruit and vegetables
* deli meats (like ham and salami)
* smoked seafood (like smoked salmon).

You can eat any of the above foods if they are cooked thoroughly, though, as this kills any bacteria present.

Food rules

To minimise your risk of listeria:

* Refrigerate food (especially meat and dairy) at less than 5 degrees Celsius.
* Wash fruit and vegetables well, under cold running water.
* Cook your foods thoroughly. Sorry, no medium–rare steak for a few months.
* Refrigerate leftover meat within an hour of cooking it.
* If you're eating leftovers, reheat until the core is 75 degrees Celsius. (And reheat in the oven or on the stovetop. Microwaves don't distribute heat evenly.)
* Store all food in sealed containers.
* When cooking, wash your hands before, during and after.

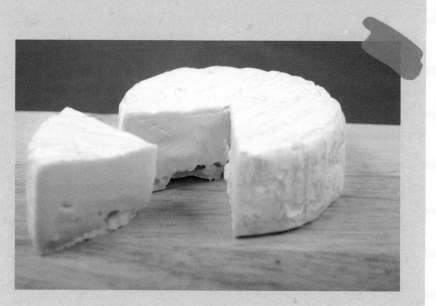

To brie or not to brie?

Interruption from an expert

Nutrition during pregnancy

If you're anything like me, the minute you fall pregnant, you get immediate cravings for Mersey Valley cheese, ice cream and literally anything that has sugar in it.

Which is fine—but.

You are also feeding another little human when you're up the duff. Even though I really, really wanted to survive on sugar and white bread (and preferably, sugar *on* white bread) throughout my pregnancies, I knew that wasn't really a great idea.

As with all things pregnancy-related, I turned to my dream team. Dr Len explained the do's and don'ts of pregnancy nutrition—and here he is to do the same for you.

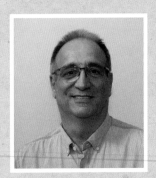

The Obstetrician
Dr Len Kliman

Why the emphasis on food during pregnancy?

Nutrition is incredibly important when you're pregnant. Not only does your body experience significant physiological changes, you also need to nourish your growing baby. There's a risk of both maternal under-nutrition (which can result in premature and underweight babies) and maternal over-nutrition (which can lead to gestational diabetes). Below are some of the most frequently asked questions in my clinic.

Should I see a dietician?

At your first antenatal visit your doctor will try to get some sort of understanding of what your diet is like. You don't need to see a dietician unless you have a pre-existing condition that might interfere with pregnancy nutrition. These include under-nutrition, obesity, diabetes and food allergies. A dietician will help you put together a food program that will meet your nutritional needs.

How much weight will I gain?

It depends on how much you weigh to begin with. If you have a body mass index (BMI) of 18 to 25, then an average weight gain in pregnancy will be somewhere between 12 and 15 kilograms. (To calculate your BMI, simply divide your weight, in kilograms, with your height in metres, squared.) If you are mildly obese with a BMI between 25 and 30, aim for a weight gain in pregnancy of somewhere between 7 and 12 kilograms. If you have a BMI of over 30, you still need to gain weight in pregnancy, but if you can limit it to 9 kilograms with sensible diet and exercise you are doing all you can do to care for your pregnancy.

How many calories do I need?

In the first trimester there is no real need to increase your caloric intake. In the second trimester, try to eat an extra 350 calories per day, and in the third trimester increase this to 450 calories a day. To put this in context, a piece of wholegrain bread is around 300 calories.

As far as actual nutrients, stick to unprocessed wholefoods as much as possible. Avoid trans fats and eat plenty of fresh fruit, vegetables and whole grains. Increase the amount of protein you eat (1.1 grams for every kilogram you weigh) and eat 175 grams of carbs daily (again, to put this in context, one piece of wholegrain bread has about 56 grams of carbs).

Do I need to take a multivitamin?

It's a good idea. Your doctor will send you off for a blood test that will check your blood count, iron stores, vitamin D levels and thyroid function in the first trimester, and again at 28 weeks, but even if all of these results are within the normal range, we recommend taking a multivitamin, such as Elevit or Blackmores Pregnancy and Breast-feeding vitamins. These contain:

* **Folate**: shown to reduce the incidence of foetal abnormalities. We recommend taking it for at least one month before you conceive, and continuing until you're at least twelve weeks along. If you've had a previous child with a neural tube defect, or you are diabetic or have a condition which interferes with folate absorption, take Megafol, which has a higher dosage of folate.
* **Vitamin B12**: Important for brain development in the developing foetus.
* **B group vitamins**: About 25 per cent of pregnant women carry a single copy of a gene which can interfere with vitamin B metabolism.
* **Vitamin D**: Vitamin D deficiency is quite common in pregnancy, and this can lead to a deficiency in your baby, which can be associated with impaired skeletal development. Most prenatal vitamins only contain a small amount of vitamin D, so if you're deficient, you'll need to take an additional supplement.
* **Calcium**: Adequate calcium intake has been shown to reduce the incidence of high blood pressure disorders in pregnancy and premature labour. While most of us will get the calcium we need from dairy products and green leafy vegetables, if you're not able to eat dairy, you'll need a calcium supplement containing 1000 milligrams per tablet.
* **Iron**: You already know pregnancy is demanding, but did you know that your growing baby could deplete your iron stores? Due to the increase in your blood volume and the demands placed by the developing foetus and placenta, it's really important to have adequate iron intake during pregnancy.

Your doctor will check your iron stores at the first antenatal visit and then again at 28 weeks' gestation. If your iron stores are found to be low, you'll be put on a supplement.

* **Iodine**: Since some women are prone to an underactive thyroid during pregnancy, iodine intake is very important (iodine is essential for making the thyroid hormone). Aim for at least 150 micrograms of iodine per day—most over-the-counter pregnancy multivitamins contain 220 micrograms per day and are therefore sufficient.

And one more don't . . .

Do not look at your vagina while pregnant!

When I was pregnant with Billie, I made the epic mistake of looking at my vagina with a mirror. What. A. Goddamn. Horror show. I remember hearing myself gasp (and I'm not a gasper!), freaking out and calling my doctor. 'Something's really wrong,' I said. 'I think my vagina is broken. It looks like all the stuff that's meant to be on the inside has come out. How do I put it back in?' After getting me to promise not to look at my vagina until about a year after I'd had the baby, Dr Len told me that it was all normal and that, eventually, everything would go back to where it came from. And it did. Thank fark.

My advice to you? Don't look. Don't be curious. Don't feel like you have to check. Trust me: you don't want to see.

Pregnancy exercise: The first trimester

As Dr Len said, continuing to exercise throughout your pregnancy is not only safe, it's fantastic for your health, and for your baby's. I loved working out during my pregnancies. Sure, some days it was a complete slog, but most of the time keeping fit made me feel strong, healthy and best of all, happy. We'll discuss pregnancy exercise in greater detail in Month 4, but for now, here's what you need to know about huffy-puffy in the first trimester.

* The first three months are crucial for your baby's healthy development, so it's important to avoid overheating. Keep cool by wearing loose clothing and having regular water breaks. Avoid exercising in hot environments and modify your workout to a low to moderate intensity. Huffing and puffing? You're pushing yourself too hard.

* Focus on your posture, core and pelvic floor muscles. This will help you better cope with your changing body. These muscles are often stretched and weakened through pregnancy, leading to back pain, poor posture and pelvic floor issues. Keeping your core strong will support your back and pelvis, plus help you to recover and return to your pre-pregnancy shape. Be aware of your pelvic floor before you start any exercise (for instance, if you're lifting a weight, be sure your pelvic floor is 'on' first). Not sure how to switch your pelvic floor on? Head to a Clinical Pilates class for a primer or see Shira's tips on page 42.

* Choose low-impact options to protect your joints and pelvic floor, which can become looser as a result of hormones that flood your body during pregnancy to prepare your body for labour. Swimming and stationary cycling are fantastic low-impact activities. Start gently and listen to your body.

Interruption from an expert

Pelvic floor exercises

Ever done that thing where you get to your front door and start doing the 'I need to do a wee' dance?

I have, and it sucks. I mean, is it too much to ask that I get to do a wee where I want, when I want?! If, like me, you'd like to avoid pissing into your daughter's nappy because you cannot bloody wait to get home and do a wee*, *do your pelvic floor exercises* (see Bec's Workouts, page 99). OK? Here I've asked my beloved Shira Kramer to explain the what and the why of pelvic floors.**

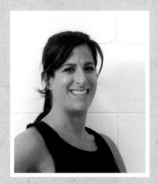

The Women's Health Physiotherapist
Shira Kramer

What's the pelvic floor?

Your pelvic floor muscles are responsible for supporting your bowel, bladder and uterus. Due to the increased weight of your baby (plus the placenta and all that extra fluid) and the effects of pregnancy hormones like relaxin (which allows your muscles and ligaments to loosen), these muscles become stretched and weakened during pregnancy. In fact, one in three women will suffer pelvic floor issues post-birth. By exercising these muscles effectively during your pregnancy, you will have better awareness of the area during labour and better continence control later.

*   Yes, I did this. I recommend the nappies from Huggies—great absorbency.
**   You're doing the exercises right now, aren't you? ***
*** Me too.

What can I do to help?

Regular pelvic floor exercises will help improve and maintain tone down below. The good news is, this is so simple to do—and of course, you can do it *anywhere*.

To do the exercise and switch on your pelvic floor, tighten and lift around your back and front passage as if you're holding on to go to the toilet. Do five lifts, three times a day. For extra credit, do one long hold (up to ten seconds) daily. Try to do the exercises at a certain time every day, so you remember—making your coffee in the morning, brushing your teeth or, my personal favourite, when you're at a red light (red light = hold tight).

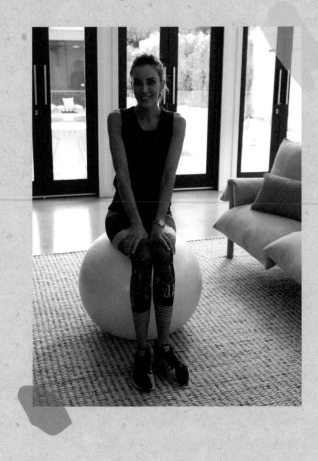

Pregnancy skincare

Apart from choosing to omit products with Vitamin A (because: retinols), my preggo beauty routine didn't change too much from my normal beauty routine. Whether I'm pregnant or not, I try to use products that contain as many natural ingredients as possible, and avoid nasty stuff like artificial preservatives, fragrances and foaming agents. Here's a quick guide to the genius products I used when I was up-duffed, and why they worked.

Preggo problem 1: Dry skin

The biggest change in my skin was how dry it became. Like, sultana-sitting-in-the-sun dry. I applied lip balm approximately every ten minutes and still, they were dry and chapped. I practically swam in Go-To Exceptionoil for eight months—it's really luxurious and the formula means the oil sinks into your skin, rather than sitting on top and feeling all greasy. In the late stages of pregnancy, Chris would rub this on me (because I couldn't move). He didn't mind because he was already shaving my legs anyway.

Preggo problem 2: Itchy skin

When I was pregnant with the twins, the skin on my tummy was stretched to the maximus. I'm talking paper thin, which made it extremely itchy. Even typing the word *itchy* now takes me back to those days when I'd be presenting the weather and trying to talk about the upcoming southerly and *all I could think about was wanting to itch my bloody belly.* Unfortunately, the absolute last thing you want to do in this situation is scratch your skin, because the skin is fragile and scratching can cause scarring. Fantastic. My dermal clinician Kirsty (who works at the fabulous Liberty skin clinic in Melbourne; tell her I sent you) advised me to rub the itchy areas with a flat hand. It was a bit like replacing my vodka soda with a soda (i.e. kind of boring and not at all the same), but it worked, because I came away completely scar-free, despite measuring 47 weeks, for a single pregnancy, the day I delivered the twins. Nope, that's not a typo. I measured 47 centimetres from the top of my belly to my pelvic bone. 47. Centimetres.

Preggo problem 3: **Stretch marks**

When your body is literally making another human, it needs to grow. And so, your skin needs to stretch. And when that happens, it can scar. Kirsty suggested I use Stratamark cream to stop stretch marks forming, and thank god I listened to her. At 31 weeks, I noticed some red, itchy marks on my belly and pointed them out to Kirsty, who immediately found me a tube of Stratamark and made me put it on that very minute.

Stratamark is a clinically proven medical product that forms a thin layer over the skin. It hydrates and protects the skin, and also helps the marks fade. Look, I'll level with you: it ain't cheap, but *it works*. I applied this to my belly multiple times a day, every day, from 31 weeks until I delivered the twins. I kid you not: I don't have stretch marks. True story. Even I cannot believe it. I mean, a stretch mark product that not only stops stretch marks forming but also fades existing ones? Where can I buy shares in this company?

Preggo problem 4: **No lasers. Boo.**

I'm a bit of a beauty junkie, and I love trying new treatments. When I'm not pregnant I love getting all sorts of laser treatments (like intense pulsed light and Laser Genesis) to make my skin look like I do not have four children. However, I wasn't comfortable doing laser treatments during pregnancy, so I indulged in milder (which were—bonus!—less painful) treatments like DermaSweep (an intense exfoliation treatment) and a HydraFacial (which infuses antioxidants and hydration into your skin) every six to eight weeks. I'd be lying if I told you I wasn't hanging out for a good zap, but while I waited, these treatments kept me from turning into that chick from *Game of Thrones* who is secretly 10,000 years old.

Preggo problem 5: **Everything hurts everywhere**

Pregnancy is great because you're incubating a tiny human life but also because you get to have massages *whenever you want them*. I used pregnancy as an excuse to get weekly massages at the divine Body Freedom Spa (South Melbourne) from 28 weeks until I delivered. These are preggo massages that are legitimately legendary. You lie on your side on a futon, with your bump supported by long pregnancy pillows. It is *so* comfortable and infinitely better than lying on your tummy with your bump hanging into a cut-out in the table, your boobs flattened by your now gigantic body. Nope. Even better, the massage is done by a qualified masseur who follows the techniques of leading UK pregnancy massage therapist Suzanne Yates. If you're not lucky enough to live in Melbourne, I suggest having your babymoon down here so you can experience one for yourself. They are *that* good.

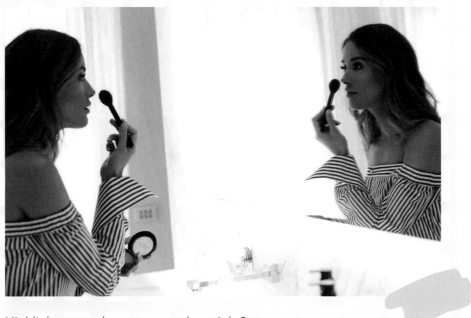

Highlighter equals pregnancy glow, right?

Your skin during pregnancy

Joanne Auld—Director of The Skincare Company and Pamper Medical Skin Clinic, Geelong—has had over 20 years' experience working in the medical and cosmeceutical industry. Here she talks about skin changes in pregnancy and how to address them.

Our hormones have such an immense impact on how our skin looks and feels, both contraception and pregnancy can really affect our skin and complexion. For women who aim to have complexion perfection, it's quite a shock when hormones play havoc with skin during and after pregnancy. During pregnancy, your skin can go through a variety of changes, including hormonal breakouts, dryness or excessive oiliness, pigmentation changes (such as melasma), the worsening of existing skin conditions (such as dermatitis), and increased sensitivity to some products, warm temperatures and sun exposure. Progesterone can increase by as much as 60 per cent, oestrogen by up to 30 per cent, and both of these have impacts on your skin. Along with keeping hydrated and getting as much rest as possible, caring for your skin with a professional skincare regime should be of utmost importance to maintain and support a healthy skin during this special time.

Although pregnancy is a breeze for some women, others can experience quite the opposite. Your skin is constantly growing and changing, so it's important to be vigilant and care for it, understanding that your previous routine may need to alter slightly. My advice would be to seek out a skincare professional for guidance.

There are some changes to your skin that require more careful attention, during and after pregnancy: these include stretch marks, melasma and rosacea.

Stretch marks

Any time your body grows quickly, you are at risk for stretch marks—the reddish, purple, pink or sometimes brown streaks (depending on your skin tone) that start to appear on your breasts, stomach, buttocks, hips and thighs. However, not every mother-to-be gets stretch marks; genetics and hormones have an impact, so if your mother or sister got stretch marks you probably will too. Once stretch marks appear they are permanent, but you can do your best to prevent them by gently exfoliating and thoroughly moisturising your bump, breasts, hips and thighs as much as you can. After birth, retinoids may help to slightly improve the stretch marks by building collagen and thickening the skin, but laser is the best option for treatment as it kick-starts the healing process.

Melasma

Melasma is a form of pigmentation thought to be stimulated by the increase in oestrogen in pregnancy. More than 50 per cent of pregnant women, especially those with darker skin, develop a 'pregnancy mask'—the darkening of pigmentation around the mouth, cheeks and forehead—and many also develop acne. Most women who have hormonal skin pigmentation tend to have olive or dark complexions. While melasma does not cause any pain or discomfort, it can be upsetting because it is highly visible. Under our harsh Australian sun, the best solution is to apply a high SPF cream and wear a wide-brimmed hat on a daily basis.

After birth, hydroquinone is the common first treatment for melasma and works by lightening the skin. The most successful topical formulation has been a combination of hydroquinone, tretinoin (a retinoid) and a topical steroid—Kligman's formula—to lighten and exfoliate the skin. Melasma often fades on its own after pregnancy but has a strong tendency to return, so maintenance treatments and prevention are essential.

Cosmetic procedures such as chemical peels, microdermabrasion, fractional laser treatment or light-based procedures, such as red or orange light LED, can also be used after birth, but please speak to your dermal expert before proceeding.

Rosacea

Rosacea is a skin condition characterised by facial redness—especially on the cheeks, around the nose and chin, and in between the brows. It is common in those with fair skin, blue eyes and Celtic origins. People with this condition are consistently red or flush easily. Other signs of rosacea include burning or stinging sensations on the face, and extremely sensitive skin. Pregnancy can exacerbate or bring out this skin condition—your blood volume almost doubles and, while this gives you a healthy glow, in some women it results in rosacea.

Rosacea may be aggravated by oil-based facial creams, sunscreen, makeup and topical steroids, though genetic, environmental and other factors are probably the root cause. Keep your face cool to reduce flushing: minimise exposure to hot or spicy foods, alcohol, hot showers, baths and warm rooms. Protect yourself from the unforgiving sun, and use light, water-based facial sunscreen on a daily basis. Switch to water- or mineral-based make-up, as it does not tend to congest the skin.

Skincare products with lots of potent anti-inflammatory ingredients, such as aloe vera, calendula, chamomile, cucumber, provitamin B5 and green tea can assist with treating rosacea. It is best to combat rosacea by combining laser treatment with a program of lifestyle changes and skin care.

Interruption from an expert

Pregnancy and beauty products
Dr Len Kliman weighs in on pregnancy beauty.

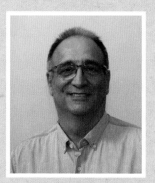

The Obstetrician
Dr Len Kliman

Can I use my beloved retinol? Pretty please?

Yes—but sparingly and not orally. Retinol, or retinoids, are a group of chemicals related to vitamin A, which has been shown to cause significant fatal abnormalities in animal trials. However, the studies used oral retinoids, not retinoids that are applied topically, on the skin. Applying retinol to the skin in small amounts, and preferably not every day, is fine.

Any other skincare chemicals to be aware of?

Salicylic acids—commonly used in acne treatment or skin peels—have been shown to cause foetal abnormalities in animal trials (taken orally, not applied to the skin). Again, if used sparingly during pregnancy, salicylic acids should be fine as the amount absorbed through your skin is minimal.

Can I dye my hair?

Yes. There's no evidence of any risk to the foetus by using routine hair dyes in pregnancy. The absorption of hair dyes through your scalp is minimal and the amount of hair dye that would be transferred across the placenta is minute and of no risk to your baby.

There has been some research to show that commercial hair dyes can cause problems, but the doses used in these studies are massive, far more than would be used in a routine hair dye. You may experience some scalp irritation due to increased sensitivity, but otherwise there's no cause for concern. Keep calm and colour on.

What about a sneaky spray tan?

Again, this is fine. The active ingredient in most spray tans is a sugar called DHA (dihydroxyacetone). It is not readily absorbed through the skin so it doesn't get in your bloodstream, meaning there's no way it will cross over to the foetus. While there haven't been any major scientific studies to back this up, tanning is not thought to be an issue because of the way the active ingredient works. Again, you may experience irritation due to increased sensitivity, but that's about it.

Do watch out for oral tanning medications (or injectables), though—these should absolutely be avoided in pregnancy.

Can I keep doing my laser hair removal? How about laser skin rejuvenation?

Yes. While there are no clinical studies to prove that laser hair removal is completely safe during pregnancy, the reality is that laser hair removal only raises the temperature of the surface of the skin—it does not affect anything deeper than the epidermis. With laser skin rejuvenation, be careful of hyperpigmentation—pregnant women are at a higher risk of this.

My go-to preggo beauty products

Disclaimer: I'm an ambassador for The Skincare Company and THE FACE by The Skincare Company. That said, I'm an ambassador because I love their products and they really, truly make me look and feel like a million bucks.

* Moisturiser (with sunscreen), *The Skincare Company*
* Daily cleanser, *The Skincare Company*
* Vitamin C serum, *The Skincare Company*
* Exfoliant serum, *The Skincare Company*
* Hyaluronic B5 serum, *The Skincare Company*
* Hydration booster, *The Skincare Company*
* Exceptionoil, *Go-To*
* Stretch mark cream, *Stratamark*
* Self-tan mousse, *Spray Aus*
* Dry shampoo, *Klorane*
* Luminous foundation, THE FACE by *The Skincare Company*
* Baked bronzer in Fiji, THE FACE by *The Skincare Company*
* Baked bronzer in satin glow (as a setting powder), THE FACE by *The Skincare Company*
* Mineral blush in nectar, THE FACE by *The Skincare Company*
* Precision eyebrow pencil in blonde, THE FACE by *The Skincare Company*
* Gel eyeliner in sienna, THE FACE by *The Skincare Company*
* Gel lipliner in ballet, THE FACE by *The Skincare Company*
* Lipstick in Angelina, THE FACE by *The Skincare Company*
* Shimmering skin perfector creme in opal by *Becca*
* Nail polishes by *Kester Black* (these polishes are chemical-free and come in amazing colours)

weeks 5-8

What's happening with baby

It's still early days, but so much is happening. Your baby's nervous system and major organs are beginning to take shape. Their heart is already beating. Tiny swellings known as 'limb buds' are forming—eventually these will become your baby's arms and legs.

At this stage, your baby is being nourished by an egg sac in your womb—the placenta hasn't quite finished developing.

What's happening with you

By week five, you'll have missed your first period, which will no doubt have you scrambling for a pregnancy test.

You might start to feel those classic preggo symptoms around now—tiredness, nausea, sore boobs. You might get some light bleeding, too—usually this is nothing to worry about, but it's always a good idea to tell your doctor or midwife.

Size-wise . . .

Your baby is on par with a kidney bean.

Month 2

Public or private?

Pretty soon, you'll have to decide whether you want to give birth as a public patient (which means your expenses will be covered by Medicare) or a private one (where you'll be out of pocket).

I was a private patient for all three births. I chose my obstetrician, Dr Len, and fell in love with him almost from the moment I met him. He was such a caring, familiar and nurturing presence, and always made me feel safe. It was important to me that I see the same doctor throughout my pregnancy, and I wanted to have a private room at the hospital when I delivered and recovered. For all these reasons, I chose to be a private patient.

When you're thinking about whether to go public or private, it's good to consider:

* Your own health. Do you have any health issues? Did you conceive easily? If you had trouble falling pregnant, perhaps an obstetrician is a better choice—someone who will know your history and be able to advise you all the way through.
* Who would you like to care for you—a midwife (as in public care), a doctor, or an obstetrician?
* Do you want to give birth at home? This is usually done by a private obstetrician or private midwife. Or would you rather go to a hospital?
* If you want private care, can you afford it? Out-of-pocket expenses can rack up to more than $5000—babies ain't cheap!

Who will look after you?

In public care, you can choose from midwives (who will see you at your pregnancy appointments, and be with you for the birth of your baby—though it is unlikely to be the same midwives all the way through), or you can have 'shared care', where you see your own GP for some appointments and midwives at your local hospital for others.

In private care, you will have your own obstetrician. If you have pregnancy risk factors or complications, this might be a better choice for you.

Where will you give birth?

Even if you're a public patient, you can still have a private room if you use private health insurance (be sure to check your private health plan—lots of insurers need you to have had pregnancy cover for up to a year before you actually introduce sperm to egg. Ridic, I know).

Many hospitals have birth centres, where minimal medical intervention (read: no drugs) is offered. You can do this as a public or private patient.

If you're a private patient, you will usually deliver at a private hospital or you can choose a private obstetrician who will deliver at a public hospital to cut down the hospital fees. Be sure your chosen obstetrician delivers at the hospital you've chosen (your hospital will have a list).

How much moolah?

If you're a public patient, all costs are covered by Medicare. (If you choose shared care, you may have to pay the gap for your GP appointments.)

Private patients will receive some money back from Medicare, but as I've said, expect to fork out at least $5000 for your obstetrician, hospital stay and other costs (like ultrasounds and blood tests). You might be eligible to get some of this money back from your healthcare fund—look into it.

Other things to know

Whether you go private or public, having a baby in Australia is extremely safe (thank our lucky stars, right?) and you should feel comfortable with whatever you choose. That said, here are a few insider tips on both.

PRIVATE:
* Appointments generally run on time, or very close to it.
* Your obstetrician will be on call for you, so you can ask any question you like, at any time of day.
* You need to book an obstetrician quite early. Preferably just after missing your first period. Failing that, as soon as you know you're pregnant, it's wise to look into finding an obstetrician in your area. You want to make sure you've got the good Doc locked down before the first trimester ends.
* Your obstetrician may not turn up to the birth. They're in high demand.

PUBLIC:

* Appointments can be hard to secure and hard to change.
* You may not see the same midwife/doctor every time.
* Appointments can run quite late.
* You'll have to book yourself into your local hospital. Some hospitals have a cut-off date when you have to have booked your bed (i.e. three months before your due date), and others don't allow you to book in until a certain time, so check this out early.

Pap smears

At your first visit, your doctor will ask you the date of your last pap smear. If you're due for one, you should have this done during early pregnancy and if you're not due, then there's no need to have another one during pregnancy.

Interruption from an expert

What the hell is happening to my body?

Being pregnant can sometimes feel like you're a human science experiment—or an actor in a horror movie. So much stuff happens to you every single day—and so much of it is beyond your control. From morning sickness (that lasts *all* day for some unlucky ladies) to varicose veins that look like they could double as tattoos, to heartburn that makes you regret everything you've ever eaten, we preggos really suffer sometimes. Ugh. Here, I've asked my obstetrician Dr Len to talk us through some of the most common pregnancy symptoms, and what you can do about them.

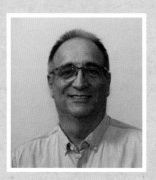

The Obstetrician
Dr Len Kliman

CONSTIPATION

What's going on: About 30 per cent of pregnant women will experience constipation. Most who suffer from it will experience it throughout their pregnancies (not just in the first trimester, for instance). Pregnant women become constipated because of the increase in the hormone progesterone, which decreases muscle tone in the bowel.

What you can do about it: Drink plenty of water and increase your fibre intake (i.e. eat lots of fresh fruits and vegetables, and wholegrains). You can also take a laxative such as Fybogel, which can help relieve symptoms.

HAEMORRHOIDS

What's going on: Another common pregnancy symptom, haemorrhoids affect around 30–40 per cent of pregnant women. Haemorrhoids are actually varicose veins that appear in your anal canal. They sometimes itch, and often hurt. Sometimes they can cause bleeding. If you don't experience haemorrhoids during pregnancy, you may experience them after labour, as the effects of pushing can pop them out.

What you can do about it: Avoid constipation, which is the main factor leading to haemorrhoids. You can also use haemorrhoid ointments. After labour, place icepacks on the area to reduce swelling. Most haemorrhoids will disappear in the weeks after labour, and surgery is rarely required.

MORNING SICKNESS

What's going on: If you're one of the 10 per cent of pregnant women who don't experience morning sickness, count yourself very lucky. Most women go through some level of nausea during pregnancy, and for an unlucky few (around 10 per cent), it persists throughout the pregnancy. While most women will feel better around the second trimester, occasionally women will be hospitalised due to morning sickness.

What you can do about it: Dietary changes are often effective. Eat small snacks rather than large meals. Eat food you know you can tolerate. For many women, this is carbs—rice, pasta, dry biscuits, toast and so on. Many women tell me that citrus-flavoured soft drinks are helpful. Avoid smells that trigger your nausea (i.e. if coffee makes you feel ill, stay away from cafes). Some women say that taking their prenatal vitamins on an empty stomach makes them feel sick. In this case, take them at the end of the day, after dinner.

You can also take medicine for morning sickness, particularly if it is so bad that you're vomiting, dehydrated or the nausea is severely impacting your daily life. See your doctor if this sounds like you—they might suggest pyridoxine or vitamin B6, both of which can help mild morning sickness. For more severe nausea, a drug like Maxolon or Zofran can be prescribed.

For very, very severe morning sickness, a hospital stay may be required. Here, you'll be put on a drip, to replace lost fluids and to administer anti-nausea medication.

STRETCH MARKS

What's going on: Stretch marks are—unfortunately—part of the deal when you're pregnant. They appear for a number of reasons. Firstly, there's a lot of mechanical stress on your skin, causing the elastic fibres to rupture, resulting in marks. Then there's the fact that your skin actually changes during pregnancy due to the increase in oestrogen. For most women, stretch marks will begin as localised swelling, which then becomes red or purple, before fading to white and then back to normal skin tone.

What you can do about it: There are plenty of creams and oils on the market to prevent stretch marks, but none have been scientifically proven. Laser treatment is the most effective solution we have at the moment. You can also use topical retinoids (after pregnancy) but these need to be used for some months to take effect.

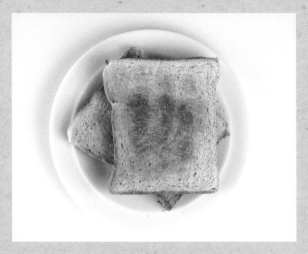

Sometimes this is all you can face . . .

ACID REFLUX

What's going on: Many women experience acid reflux or indigestion from the first trimester onwards. Some women feel it as upper abdominal discomfort, for others it's a burning feeling in the chest, and for others still, acid actually does come back up into their mouths. Not ideal, as you can imagine. The reason pregnant women experience acid reflux is because when pregnant, the valve that normally prevents reflux doesn't work very well, probably due to an increase in progesterone. The good news is that this usually goes away very quickly after labour.

What you can do about it: Take over-the-counter medications like Gaviscon, Mylanta or Zantac. If these don't work, consult your GP or physician.

VARICOSE VEINS

What's going on: Many pregnant women get varicose veins because of the increased blood volume circulating during pregnancy, and the increased pressure on the lower limbs. Some women also experience varicose veins near their vulva, called vulvar varices. These can cause swelling and aching near the opening of the vagina, and are quite difficult to treat during pregnancy. The good news is that they usually disappear quite quickly after labour.

What you can do about it: For veins on your legs, limit your time standing in the one spot as much as possible. Lie down on your side with your legs elevated as often as you can. Wear compression stockings (which help with swelling and aching).

For vulvar varices, you can wear supportive garments and apply cold compresses to relieve the pain.

So . . . you're having more than one baby

Remember how I said that when I found out I was pregnant with Oscar my first thought was: *fuuuuuuuck*?

Yeah. Imagine what I thought when I found out I was having twins.

Fucketty fuck fuck fuck. Fuck squared times a million.

I fell pregnant with Tom and Darcy not too long before we left for a wedding in South Africa. I'd been feeling really off, and wondered if I might be pregnant—we'd been trying. I weed on yet another stick and—lo and behold!—I was preggers. Again!

The thing about this wee stick was that I had weed on it super early—like, a week after we'd had sex. But those two lines showed up fierce and bold. There was no mistaking it: I was pregnant.

Chris and I were so excited. Three kids. It was perfect. I started thinking about names and the nursery and digging out Oscar's and Billie's old onesies. I had my eight-week scan and everything was normal. Another healthy baby—how bloody lucky was I?

At my eleven-week scan, I saw this weird blob on the ultrasound above the baby. Having experienced lots of ultrasounds before and kind of knowing my way around them in an amateurish way, I knew that this blob seemed out of place. It was too early in my pregnancy for it to be a placenta of that size . . . so what the hell was it?

'What's that blob there?' I asked my obstetrician, Dr Len. He smiled at me in this really odd way.

'What?' I asked, feeling anxious. He smiled some more. A kind of wry, mischievous, chuffed smile. The kind of smile your kid gives you when you've told them they cannot have any more chocolate, but they're holding a chocolate bar behind their back, just waiting for you to look away so they can get into it.

'It's another kid,' he said. 'See that?'

I looked. I saw Len move the ultrasound position to better show the 'blob' . . . and before my very eyes it materialised into *another kid*.

And it kicked and waved.

And I screamed.

'That's a baby,' he said, pointing at the first heartbeat. 'And that's another baby.'

I screamed some more. *Oh my god. Oh my god.* I believe my next words were, 'You have got to be shitting me.'

Reader, he wasn't.

I sat there in shock, sweating and shaking, and made Dr Len call Chris to tell him our news. I heard several thousand f-bombs being dropped down the line. So we were in agreement, then: having twins was crazy.

On my way out—still dazed—I ran into my midwife, Cath. She'd heard me screaming and had come to see me. 'Is everything OK?' she asked. She was worried I'd lost the baby. I couldn't muster any words other than, 'Twins.'

'Oh my god!' she said. OMG indeed.

This was pretty much everyone's reaction (except for the tabloid newspapers and social media, who asked very helpful things like, 'How is she going to carry twins? She looks like a twelve-year-old!' Charming). My mum screamed. My sister screamed. A close friend summed it up when he said, 'Oh mate. I know this is when I'm supposed to say I'm excited for you, but . . . what a fucking disaster.'

Later we found out that, during the first scan, one of the boys was 'hiding' behind the other. This is actually pretty common in the first scan with twins. Isn't that fun?

Oddly enough, I think I'd had a premonition (stay with me!) that something weird was happening. The night we conceived the twins, I had this horrible nightmare that I was pregnant and something went wrong. Of course, at that stage, I didn't even know I was pregnant—but I had this sense that something was happening, and it wasn't quite right. When I found out we were having twins, I thought, *That was it. That was the weird feeling.*

At first, I was completely freaked out about having twins. The whole thought of looking after two babies at the same time—I mean, how did people do it? It was hard enough caring for one. Two? How would that even work?

I also worried that I wouldn't have enough love to give. My heart was already so full with love for Chris, Oscar and Billie. Was there room for two more people in there? I had no idea.

My twin pregnancy

Being pregnant with the twins was completely different to my other pregnancies. I used to wonder what other women were talking about when it came to morning sickness; I'd just never experienced it. Then I fell pregnant with Darcy and Tom and . . . whoa. The most innocuous smells made me gag. Foods I loved completely turned me off. I didn't throw up, but I gagged a lot. Again, such fun times.

I thought I'd been tired with the first two pregnancies, but this was something else altogether. I was exhausted basically from day one. When I was seven weeks pregnant, we went to Cape Town, South Africa, for a friend's wedding. I thought I must have had the worst case of jet lag ever—I just couldn't move from the couch or my bed. I felt like I'd stayed up all night and then run a marathon. And then done it all over again. I felt like this every day, for the entire length of my pregnancy.

Later, my ribs began to stretch and flare to accommodate the boys growing inside me. It felt like I had a very sharp knife permanently jammed into my cartilage, twisting every so often to loosen up the ribs. It was absolutely excruciating. I started googling things like, 'wheelchairs in Melbourne' and 'how soon can I go on bed rest?'

At week 28, I started using a pair of Chris's old crutches to walk around—the boys were getting big, and were starting to move down. Imagine holding up a 10-kilo weight with your fist—all day, every day. That's what it feels like to be pregnant with twins. But instead of holding them up with your fist, you're holding them up with your vagina. Luckily I didn't need to use the crutches for more than a few days—I had some very intense physio and did Pilates—but by the end of the pregnancy, I was carrying my belly whenever I walked (which, admittedly, was not too often by that stage). You know how Baby carries a watermelon in *Dirty Dancing*? That was me. Every single day.

If I haven't made being pregnant with twins sound excruciating enough, my stomach also stretched so much that you could almost see *through* my skin. The skin was so tight that you could see veins appearing all over it. I looked like Ripley from *Alien*.

Interruption from an expert

Tests, tests, tests

We've all dreamed about our first pregnancy ultrasound—hearing the *ba-boom ba-boom* of the speedy heartbeat, seeing the flutter of the tiny little being inside us. But in addition to this lovely milestone is a battery of other tests you'll do early in your pregnancy—and sometimes, later—to make sure both you and baby are healthy and well.

Dr Len explains everything you need to know about pregnancy tests.

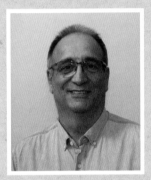

The Obstetrician
Dr Len Kliman

What happens in the first visit?

At your first antenatal visit—essentially, the first time you see your obstetrician or GP when you find out you're pregnant— your doctor will ask you for a full medical and surgical history. It's important to know if you have any medical conditions that may affect you during your pregnancy, or need to be addressed.

At your first visit, you'll undergo a range of blood tests:

* **Full blood examination:** This is a test of your haemoglobin to exclude anaemia and a genetic blood disorder called thalassemia. If thalassemia is suspected, a more specific test will need to be carried out.

* **Blood group and antibody screen:** It's important your doctor knows what blood type you are. Some blood types require a different level of care during pregnancy.

* **Rubella antibody status:** Most Australian women are immunised against rubella in high school. But if you are not

immune, you'll need to have the vaccination after your baby is born and avoid contact with anyone with proven rubella.

* **Syphilis serology**: This is very rarely positive but is a recommended routine test so that, in the rare instance of a positive finding, appropriate treatment can be given to protect the foetus.
* **Mid-stream urine**: This is to identify any silent infection or any previously undiagnosed kidney disease.
* **HIV**: This is to exclude this virus in pregnancy; should the test be positive, treatment can be given to limit the chance of transfer of the virus to the foetus during the pregnancy.
* **Hepatitis B serology**: If you're found to be a carrier of hepatitis B, you'll undergo preventive treatment to avoid transfer of the virus to the foetus.
* **Hepatitis C serology**: Again, it's very unlikely you carry this, but we like to be sure. If you're found to have hepatitis C, we can take certain precautions to prevent transfer of the virus to the foetus.
* **Varicella serology**: Most pregnant women are immune to chickenpox, but if you're not, we do recommend vaccinating after your baby is born.
* **Ferritin levels**: This is a measure of the stores of iron in your bloodstream. It gives us an indication of whether or not you require further iron supplementation.
* **Vitamin D levels**: Again, this tells us whether or not you need to be given additional vitamin D supplementation during the pregnancy.
* **TSH levels**: TSH is a thyroid function test and is primarily taken to ensure you don't have an underactive thyroid gland, which may need to be treated during the pregnancy.

The risks of having twins

Twins should come with their own dictionary; there are so many new words to learn when it comes to multiples. From my very first appointment, it was *dizygotic* this and *monozygotic* that. I was hearing the words, but not really understanding them. I thought I had a handle on pregnancy—but carrying twins was something very different, I was beginning to discover.

For a start, I learned that identical twins are very high risk because they share a placenta. The twins you 'want' (for lack of a better term) are non-identical twins in their own amniotic sacs. When twins share an amniotic sac or placenta, the risk of miscarrying one or both is much higher. There's also the risk of twin-to-twin transfusion syndrome (for more on this, see Month 3, page 82).

At thirteen weeks, I had a scan to see if I was carrying identical twins. First, we scanned for the sex . . . and discovered that I was having two boys. I saw one willy (yep, you can see them!) and thought, 'Please, please let the other one be a girl'—and then, we saw another willy. Two boys it was.

I felt a dread come over me, somehow knowing that the twins would be identical. Dr Ngu scanned . . . and told me there was only one placenta. Identical twin boys. Whoa. 'You and I are going to be seeing a lot more of each other,' he said. I just nodded, still dazed from the news.

From then on, I had a scan every two weeks. I was lucky: every time I had an ultrasound, Dr Ngu would say, 'They're doing beautifully. They're the same size. The placenta is doing its job perfectly.' It was a huge relief.

Interruption from an expert

Multiple pregnancy

So. Twins. Or triplets. Or—gulp—quadruplets. Geez—and you thought it was weird to have *one* other person inside you. The day I found out I was having Tom and Darcy, my world—and me, to be fair—just about keeled over. But once I armed myself with information about the twins growing inside me, I felt so much calmer. Dr Andrew Ngu explains everything you need to know about multiples—including how the hell they actually get made.

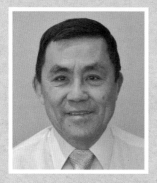

The Ultrasound Expert
Dr Andrew C.C. Ngu

How the hell do we even make twins?

There are two types of twin pregnancy—non-identical and identical twins. Non-identical twins can run in families—if you had a mother or sister who had non-identical twins, your chance is increased threefold. Non-identical twins result from two eggs being fertilised, so each foetus has its own separate genetic make-up. In every pregnancy there is an outer sac (chorionic sac) and an inner sac (amniotic sac). Non-identical twin pregnancies are in separate chorionic and amniotic sacs, each with their own placenta.

Identical twins develop as a result of the splitting of one embryo into two. Each foetus has the same genetic make-up and shares one placenta. In identical twins the two foetuses share an outer sac and may have their own inner sac. If they have their own inner sac, they are known as monochorionic diamniotic (MCDA) twins. When twins share the same inner sac as well, it is a monochorionic monoamniotic (MCMA) twin pregnancy. Identical twins do not run in the family.

weeks 9–13

What's happening with baby

At twelve weeks, your baby is actually fully formed—it just needs to grow. Their face is forming, including their eyes, which will have some pigment.

Your baby's heart is beating a crazy 180 times a minute—around two to three times faster than yours or mine. Your baby will start moving now, too, though you won't feel it for a while yet.

What's happening with you

During this month, you might start to feel moody or grumpy—this is totally normal and usually goes away pretty quickly. Since your uterus is about the size of a lime, you may also see a small bump beginning—how exciting!

Size-wise . . .

Your baby is the size of a lime. Which would go so great in that vodka soda you're craving. I know, mate. I know.

Month 3

How to style your bump

There are lots (and lots) of cool things about pregnancy, but chief among them (I reckon, anyway) is that you not only have an excuse to shop for teeny socks and adorable onesies, but also an excuse to go shopping for you—after all, your body is going to change shape (if it hasn't begun already) and you'll need *something* to wear for the next six—or maybe seven—months.

When I was pregnant with Oscar, I was adamant that I wouldn't buy too many maternity clothes. I honestly didn't think I'd need them. I'd just unbutton my jeans when they got too tight! And wear looser tops and dresses. Mmm. Not quite.

The thing is, pregnancy doesn't just mean you grow a bump: your hips widen, your boobs blow up, you get bigger all over (it's only temporary, but trust me—it happens). So all those maternity labels? They exist for a reason.

After three pregnancies, I feel like I've learned quite a bit about maternity dressing. Here are my top tips:

* **Maintain your own style:** Are you a preppy dresser? Sporty? A little boho? There's maternity clothing out there that will meet your needs. There's no need to compromise on your own unique style just because you're carrying a little extra someone.

* **Experiment:** OK, I know I said you should maintain your style. But for some women, pregnancy can be a time of experimenting. Lots of women I know wouldn't normally wear bodycon dresses or denim overalls—but while pregnant, it felt fun and fresh to wear stuff like this. So have a bit of fun with it, too.

* **Shop your own wardrobe:** Chances are, you'll have some long, loose, draped tops or dresses you can still wear while preggo. Stretchy stuff is great, too—leather leggings, normal leggings, jersey tops and dresses all look and feel great.

* **Denim heaven:** Invest in at least one great pair of maternity jeans, no matter the weather. I bought mine from ASOS (Topshop do a good version, too) and I still wear them now, they're so comfy. Jeans can be styled up or down, so you'll never have that awful dilemma of having 'nothing' to wear.

* **Go elastic:** For pants, look for elastic waists. Elastic is your friend. As are potato chips.
* **Avoid seams:** With dresses and tops, avoid seams that run down your tummy—they will ride up and make your belly look weird. I bought this beautiful loose yellow tent dress when I was pregnant and I was so excited to wear it . . . until I tried it on and saw that there was a giant seam running down the middle of my belly. It looked so wrong.
* **Ditch the underwire:** If you're anything like me, your boobs will start to explode pretty much the second the sperm says hello to the egg. Invest in some maternity bras. These bras are still supportive (necessary) but don't have underwire (which can press into the breast and maybe cause mastitis). Most of them can also be used for nursing later on.
* **Don't forget your swimwear and activewear:** I loved swimming when I was pregnant. I wore my normal bikinis, or went a size up to accommodate my growing boobs. ASOS and Topshop do great maternity swimwear—both bikinis and one-pieces. For activewear, choose a good pair of compression tights (which help with circulation) and a good sports bra. I've listed some brands on page 72 that I love.
* **Treat yourself, later:** Straight talk: you will absolutely get sick of your maternity wardrobe by the 39th week. Probably even earlier than that. And you'll probably grow out of a lot of it, too—when I was pregnant with the twins, I was down to one pair of pants and two tops that I could fit into by the end. It was like *Groundhog Day*, except not as funny. Because I couldn't wear what I wanted, I 'treated' myself by going online and looking at clothes I knew I'd be able to wear soon after having my babies. I kept a little bookmark folder of all the lovely things I knew I could buy soon, and it kept me sane.

Maternity labels I love:

* ASOS Maternity (especially great for jeans—they come in different lengths and have an amazingly comfortable stretchy waistband)
* Bae the Label (the chicest maternity wear on the planet)
* Bonds (they do great, affordable maternity bras, nursing bras and underwear that's made to fit your growing bump)
* Hello Monday (this new Aussie label does great maternity sportswear—if you need to go up a size for your sports bra, try them. They also do activewear for nursing mums, with tops that are supportive and clip up and down, and high-waisted tights for exercising after your pregnancy)
* Husk
* Jaggad (full disclosure: I co-own this brand. But I co-own it for a reason—we make excellent activewear)
* Kmart (for excellent, cheap maternity bras)
* Kookai (again, not strictly maternity, but their fabrics are stretchy and comfortable—perfect for growing bumps)
* Legoe (great for long, stretchy dresses)
* Seed (not strictly a maternity brand, but they do lots of loose, drapey clothing that works for preggos)
* Soon Maternity

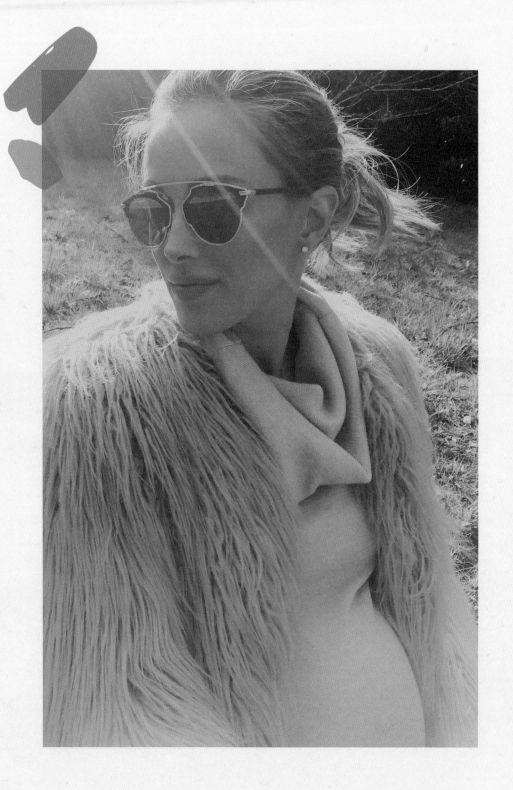

Interruption from an expert

Genetic testing

By now, your doctor has probably told you all about the tests you'll need to do as a pregbot. One of the most important tests you'll do while pregnant is genetic testing, which is done in the first trimester. Genetic tests screen for abnormalities in the chromosomes that can indicate hereditary issues. Some are common and not problematic, while others require more attention. Dr Len is here again to explain exactly what it all means.

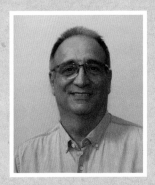

The Obstetrician

Dr Len Kliman

What do genetic tests check for?

While genetic testing is not compulsory, there are two basic tests that are offered to all pregnant women. If you have them, they're carried out at about ten weeks' gestation.

The first is genetic carrier screening, a test to ensure you don't carry a faulty gene you could pass on to your foetus. These include genes associated with cystic fibrosis, fragile X syndrome and spinal muscular atrophy.

The second genetic screen is cell-free DNA testing, a test for conditions where the foetus carries an extra chromosome. These are called trisomy conditions. Trisomy 21 is Down syndrome but the test also ensures that the foetus does not have an extra number 13, 18, 15 or 16, or abnormalities of the sex chromosomes X and Y.

If your results for either of these tests is positive, you'll receive genetic counselling and a full briefing of your options going forward.

Finding out the sex

As with most things during pregnancy, everyone has an opinion on whether you should find out the sex of your baby.

Want to know what I think? You do whatever you damn well please. It's your baby. (And if anyone asks why you're finding out—or not—feel free to tell them exactly that. 'Because it's my baby. Not yours.')

With Oscar, Chris and I were desperate to find out the sex. We just couldn't help ourselves. The excitement of being unexpectedly pregnant made us really inquisitive—and we also wanted to plan and organise as much as we possibly could. For some reason, I always thought I would have a girl first, so it was a huge—pleasant—surprise to discover that I was pregnant with a boy. When my doctor said, 'It's a boy,' I said, 'What? Are you sure? You'd better check again.' He—very calmly—told me that unless Oscar had three legs, he was definitely a boy.

Because I had always imagined having girl babies, finding out Oscar was a boy made me feel like I'd won the baby lottery. I'm so happy we found out the sex because it meant that for the rest of my pregnancy I was on cloud nine (when I wasn't feeling my abs separate from each other or drowning my feelings in mint choc chip ice cream).

With Billie, Chris and I decided to leave the sex a surprise. We wanted to do things a little differently, and knew that whoever ended up exiting my vag would be beautiful and absolutely beloved, no matter their sex. However, one day, around twenty weeks or so, I was having a routine ultrasound when the midwife doing the scan suddenly pointed the wand over what looked like a giant hamburger on its side. 'Oh my god!' I said. 'That is a vagina.' She looked terrified, as she knew I didn't want to know, and we both agreed that she wouldn't confirm or deny it . . . but I know a vag when I see one, and I had *definitely* seen one. I was so confident that I started ordering furniture for a girl's nursery.

And with the twins, we found out the sex as soon as we could. A twin pregnancy is overwhelming enough as it is—we wanted to know as much as possible, so we could plan our lives. I did not need any extra surprises at that point. And even though I'd been surprised with the sexes both times before,

I still wasn't prepared when the doctor told me I was housing two identical boys in there. Boys. Three boys. Where were all those girls I'd dreamed of? Isn't it funny what life throws at you?

If you want to find out the sex . . .

You'll have an ultrasound at around 19–20 weeks where you can find out the sex of your baby. You can now find out earlier than this—at around ten weeks—with a new test called the non-invasive prenatal test (NIPT), which is a blood test that looks for genetic abnormalities and can also determine the sex.

And if you don't . . .

Tell every ultrasound technician you see in advance, just in case they accidentally say something.

Forget about the giant sideways hamburger image. Now that I've told you, you'll be looking out for it. If you don't want to know, don't look!

What to say when people say, 'Oh, why did you find out the sex? Don't you want a surprise?'

'No. Now bugger off.'

What to say when people say, 'Oh, why don't you find out the sex? Don't you want to know?'

'No. Now bugger off.'

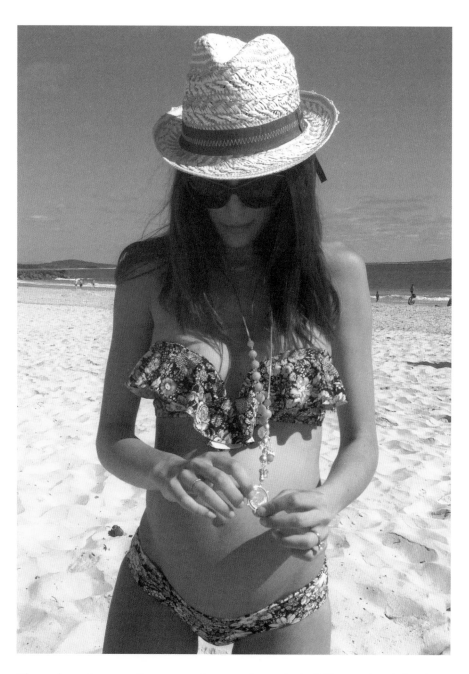

The only real way to figure out the sex of your baby? Um . . . by delivering it. No strings. No rings. Soz, Greek grandmas of the world.

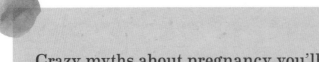

Crazy myths about pregnancy you'll probably hear along the way

When your bump starts to show, a funny thing happens: all people can talk to you about is the baby. Which is fun and exciting . . . but can also get a bit weird, especially when they start telling you that you're 'definitely' having a boy because of how your tummy looks (seriously, ten seconds later someone will say you're 'definitely' having a girl for the exact same reason). There are plenty of crazy myths about pregnancy . . . here are some of the weirder ones I've heard.

* You have to be upside down or lie with your feet up after sex to get pregnant. (Trust me on this one: no.) Also, lying down after sex helps the semen 'marinate'. Sorry, no. (Also, now you have the words 'semen' and 'marinate' in your head. Sorry about that.)

* Got heartburn? Your baby has thick hair, apparently. (Oh, and the extra hair is causing your heartburn. Makes sense.)

* Want to know your baby's sex? Oh, there are plenty of ways, apparently. Craving sweet foods? That's a girl. Carrying low? That's a boy. If you want a really definitive answer, just attach a ring to a piece of string, lie down and have someone hang the ring-string over your belly. If it swings anticlockwise, you've got a girl on your hands, clockwise and you've got a boy.

* Baby in a breach position? No problem. Just hold a torch to Mum's vag—the baby will turn its head towards the light.

* Want to go into labour? Drink raspberry leaf tea. Take a spoonful of castor oil. (Ugh. No, thank you.) Eat pineapples. Have a spicy curry. Drink red wine. (OK, that one I can get down with.) Do squats. (No way.) Go for a long walk. (Sod off.) Or my favourite . . . have sex! Because every woman who has a four-kilogram person inside her wants another person inside her, right?

Spoiler alert: these are all bullshit.

Interruption from an expert

Twelve-week ultrasound (and other tests)

There's nothing quite like seeing your first ultrasound. While it doesn't look like a baby yet—just a fluttering heartbeat—it's mind-blowing to imagine the little life inside you. Ultrasounds make pregnancy feel very real, in an amazing way.

I was lucky enough to have Dr Andrew Ngu perform my ultrasounds. I've asked him a few questions to get the lowdown on the scans you need, and why you need them.

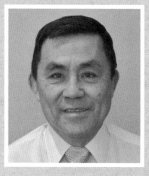

The Ultrasound Expert
Dr Andrew C.C. Ngu

When will I have ultrasounds?

Most women will be offered screening ultrasounds once in each trimester: at 12–13 weeks, 20–22 weeks (see page 120 in Month 5) and then at 30–36 weeks (see page 177 in Month 7).

What happens at the first ultrasound?

The first trimester ultrasound can be performed internally (i.e. with a wand that is inserted into your vagina) and/or through your abdomen—think of every Hollywood movie you've ever seen about pregnancy. Usually, when the pregnancy is closer to six weeks, transvaginal ultrasounds are more accurate. At thirteen weeks, most ultrasounds can be performed transabdominally, although transvaginal ultrasounds provide better images as the foetus is closer to the ultrasound probe. However, it is less elegant.

In your first ultrasound, we'll be checking that you have a healthy, ongoing pregnancy in the uterus and determining how old the pregnancy is (the gestational age). We also check for the number of foetuses, and in the case of multiples, the type of twins (or other). After eleven weeks or so we can also check for some abnormalities and assess the likelihood of chromosomal abnormalities such as Down syndrome.

How do you figure out how old the foetus is?

We measure the length of the crown of the head to the rump (we call this the crown–rump length, or CRL). It's accurate to within five days. It's really important to know the age of the pregnancy, and the first trimester ultrasound is the most accurate time to figure this out. We want to know how old the foetus is so we can do other tests (like blood tests) at the right time, and also assess the proper growth of the foetus as your pregnancy progresses. It'll also help later in your pregnancy, if you are deemed to be overdue and need an induction.

Some women have bleeding or pain during their first trimester. Can an ultrasound check what's going on?

Bleeding can occur in up to 40 per cent of pregnancies in the first trimester. Understandably, this can create a lot of anxiety. In most cases, the cause of the bleeding is unknown but it could be due to an adverse pregnancy outcome—such as a failed pregnancy or pregnancy 'outside' the uterus (such as ectopic pregnancy, where the pregnancy is in the fallopian tube, not the uterus). An ultrasound examination allows early diagnosis and management of complications—this can also reassure most pregnant women that all is well with their pregnancy.

Pain in the pelvis is another common symptom in early pregnancy and again, it makes women very anxious. It can be associated with bleeding. In the majority of cases, pain is due to the uterus expanding to house the pregnancy and the associated changes in the ligaments supporting the uterus. However, if you are worried, and particularly if there is bleeding, you should inform your obstetrician. An ultrasound may rule out a pregnancy in the fallopian tube, a cyst in the ovaries or fibroid in the uterus.

What about testing for Down syndrome and other genetic abnormalities?

There are screening and diagnostic tests available to detect Down syndrome in pregnancy. A screening test is performed at 10½–13 weeks to work out the chance of Down syndrome, and there is also a more accurate diagnostic test, which will say for sure if the condition is present in the foetus. The chance of having a foetus with Down syndrome increases with the age of the mother.

There are two types of screening tests available. These are:

1. A combined blood test and an ultrasound scan. The blood test is taken from ten weeks and three days to thirteen weeks, and the ultrasound is performed from eleven weeks and three days to thirteen weeks and six days. It is very important that the tests are done at this correct time. The combined test can detect up to 90 per cent of Down syndrome pregnancies. You'll be given a risk ratio—for example, one in 15,000, one in 1000. A risk of more than one in 300 chances is considered to be an increased risk.

2. The NIPT (non-invasive prenatal test) is a blood test that can be done from ten weeks and five days onwards. This test analyses the genetic material in the mother's blood and can figure out the chance of having Down syndrome and other chromosomal abnormalities. This test is a little more expensive than the combined test, but it can detect up to 99 per cent of Down syndrome pregnancies.

With both of these tests, if the risk of having Down syndrome is high, you'll then have a more accurate diagnostic test. Again, there are two types of diagnostic tests. These are:

1. **Chorionic villus sampling (CVS)**: This can be done from ten weeks, and consists of obtaining a sample from the placenta.

2. **Amniocentesis**: This can be done from sixteen weeks, and involves taking a sample from your amniotic fluid.

Both of these tests are very accurate in determining the genetic make-up of the foetus and can detect Down syndrome with 100 per cent accuracy. However, it's important to know that carrying out these tests has a small risk of losing the pregnancy—about one in 150 in CVS and one in 300 in amniocentesis.

OK! That's a lot of info.

It is. There's a second trimester ultrasound, too—but let's talk about that when we get there, OK?

What if I'm having twins?

If you're pregnant with twins, you'll be seeing your ultrasound technician a lot more regularly.

If you have non-identical twins, your ultrasounds will check to ensure that the two foetuses are growing normally (and equally) throughout the pregnancy. Usually ultrasound scans are performed every four weeks from 24 weeks onwards (unless the growth is below average in any of the scans—then more frequent scans are necessary).

In identical twins, there is also the added potential complication of twin-to-twin transfusion syndrome (TTTS), where blood may disproportionately flow from one twin (the donor) to the other twin (the recipient). This causes the donor twin to have decreased blood volume, which in turn leads to slower growth and decreased urine output. The recipient twin on the other hand is overloaded with blood, leading to increased urine output, and the increased blood volume may put extra strain on the heart causing heart failure. TTTS can occur in up to one in five identical twins and it can occur any time during the pregnancy. It can only be detected by ultrasound. So for identical twins, we perform ultrasounds every two weeks, beginning at 16–18 weeks (until 32–34 weeks) to look for signs of TTTS, in addition to checking the growth of each foetus. Luckily, if TTTS is detected, it can be treated by laser surgery.

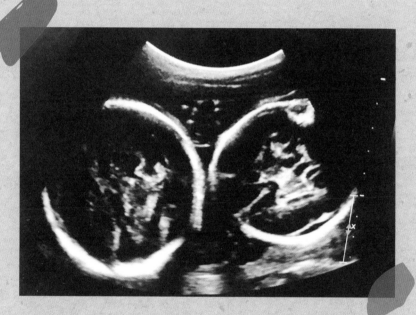

The twins

weeks 14–17

What's happening with baby

You might want to sit down for this: your baby now has fingerprints. Crazy but true.

   During this month, your baby can start to hear, and even register bright light through the lining of the womb. Your baby's sex has now been determined, too—so when you go for your ultrasound around week 20 you can check (if that's your thing).

What's happening with you

Your morning sickness is probably (hopefully) fading. Because you're getting bigger, though, you may still need to head to the loo more often (but just to wee, not to vom— silver linings and all that).

   Around this time, some women report having a higher sex drive, while other women report wanting to curl up under a doona watching *Real Housewives* marathons and eating cheese Twisties for the remainder of their pregnancies.

Size-wise . . .

Your bub is the size of an avo.

Month 4

Dude, where's my abs?

By now, your body is probably starting to change. Your boobs are probably bigger. You might have put on some weight, or even have a bump. You might have noticed that your feet start to swell at the end of the day. All normal. Carry on.

When I fell pregnant with Oscar, I expected all of this to happen, and it did: my boobs began to grow practically the minute I took the pregnancy test, and I could see my hips widening week by week. But something else happened, too. Something common, but not normal: my abs began to separate.

It sounds like I'm exaggerating—like, really Bec? Your abs *separated*? Sure—but I can tell you: they really did. This is no exaggeration.

I first noticed the separation when I was nineteen weeks pregnant with Oscar. I went to sit up from a lying position in bed and noticed that my bump turned into a bit of a pyramid as I moved—sort of like a Toblerone erupting in the middle of my tummy. Not only did this look freaky AF, it felt weird, too, as if the muscles were weak and I didn't have much control over the area. Over time, things got worse: the separation stretched even further until it felt like there was a knife wedged between my abs, which in turn, made them feel as though they were on fire. And not in, like, an Instagram emoji fire way.

Luckily, I had been pre-warned by Shira, my women's health physio, that this might happen. As soon as I noticed my Toblerone tummy, I went to her for an assessment. She diagnosed diastasis of the rectus abdominus muscle (DRAM), or abdominal separation, and prescribed me a Tubigrip compression garment to wear for the remainder of my pregnancy. She also developed a DRAM-focused prenatal exercise and Clinical Pilates program specifically for my condition. Though I couldn't avoid diastasis recti completely (I already had it by that stage), Shira's help meant that I was doing everything I possibly could to stop my DRAM causing other health issues. This resulted in pretty cruisey pregnancies with Oscar and Billie and, amazingly, no long-term health problems, even after carrying twins. I was so lucky to be educated and treated for DRAM during all three of my pregnancies—I shudder to think what kind of shape I might have been in had I not.

Interruption from an expert

All about diastasis recti

Shira Kramer breaks down how your abs, um, break down.

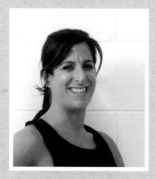

The Women's Health Physiotherapist
Shira Kramer

What's diastasis recti?

Diastasis recti, or abdominal separation (DRAM), is one of the most common conditions that I see in pregnant and postnatal patients. DRAM is the pulling apart of the long muscle and connective tissue in the middle of your abdominal wall that occurs during pregnancy or birthing.

Holy moly. What causes it?

Lots of things: abdominal weakness, hormonal changes, weight gain and the stretching of the abdominal wall can be contributing factors, as well as the pressure of pushing during delivery.

OK. How do I stop it from happening to me?

First, avoid activities that work the outer abdominals from the early stages of pregnancy. That means no sit-ups, planks or high-impact activities such as running and jumping. Also, avoid heaving up from a lying position to sitting or standing. Instead, roll onto your side first. In the mornings, pop your legs over the edge of the bed and then sit up by pushing through your arms from a sideways position. That's a good idea for all pregnant women (and new mums), whether they have a separation or not. Also, avoid excessive coughing, constipation and heavy lifting (toddlers included here!). And of course, getting started on some deep abdominal and pelvic floor muscle exercises will ensure your core and back are in good condition.

How do I know I have it?

In most cases, women don't realise they have abdominal separation until they are assessed by a medical consultant or a women's health physiotherapist. If you think you might have DRAM, look for signs of a severe abdominal separation, such as a triangle-shaped protrusion down your belly—this will look like a bulge in the centre of the abdomen, particularly when curling forward. Persistent back pain, pelvic girdle pain, a hernia or a protrusion may be indicators of a persistent separation and should be assessed by a women's health physio for treatment.

What if I have it? Is there any way to 'stitch' my abs back together?

Yes, absolutely. By looking after your abdominals during pregnancy and the early months after childbirth, the separation should resolve within about six weeks post-delivery. But there can be cases where the gap is slow to close—up to a year, or even longer. This typically happens when mothers give birth to large babies, or multiples.

I think that all pregnant women and new mothers—with or without DRAM—should see a women's health physiotherapist to monitor their separation. A physio will be able to prescribe you specific exercises and offer you an appropriate abdominal muscle support (compression garment).

What if I have DRAM but I never knew about it?

This happens, and it's not great. If left untreated, DRAM can have all sorts of nasty implications—pelvic floor dysfunction (which occurs in 66 per cent of patients with DRAM), back and pelvic girdle pain, and hernias. This may be a factor in persistent postnatal lumbar, pubic symphysis and sacroiliac pain, and even incontinence, due to the interaction of the pelvic floor and abdominal musculature as part of the core. It's never too late to do something about it.

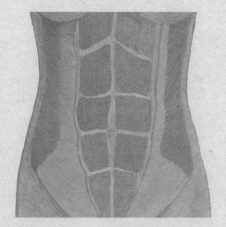 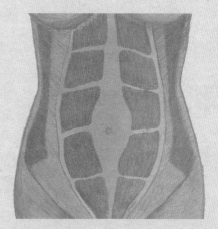

Normal abdomen   *Diastasis recti*

You can see the separation of the abdominal muscles and connective tissues in diastasis recti in the diagram on the right.

Pregnancy exercise: The second trimester

For me, staying fit during my pregnancies was a high priority. Fit, strong, healthy mums get through the rigours of pregnancy—not to mention labour and the first few months of motherhood—with greater ease and recover more efficiently.

But pregnancy can be a tricky time for a woman as she watches her body grow and change at an incredible rate. Hips get wider. Boobs get bigger. Tummies pop out. Feet hold more water than the Great Barrier Reef. It's enough to make you wonder whether your body will ever get back to its pre-baby state. I thought about this often, particularly when I was pregnant with the twins—my body felt truly alien to me (because I actually looked like one!). And even though exercise was sometimes the very, very last thing I wanted to do, I knew that if I stayed on top of my fitness, I would feel better during pregnancy, and bounce back quicker afterwards, too.

Now that you're getting a little larger, there are a few things to keep in mind during exercise.

* After sixteen weeks, avoid lying on your back—this can reduce the oxygen supply to your baby. You can modify exercises where you lie down to seated or upright positions, or a kneeling position (on your hands and knees).
* Pay special attention to strengthening your postural muscles in your upper back and core. Aim to sit tall with length in your spine, shoulders back and down.
* Avoid motionless standing—it can slow down circulation. Modify your weight training from a standing position to sitting.

Exercising during my three pregnancies

When I was pregnant with Oscar, and then Billie, I did Clinical Pilates and prenatal exercise classes a couple of times a week. I was monitored closely by Shira and her team at BeActive Physio and wore a prescribed Tubigrip compression bandage on my belly when my abdominals began to separate. One thing that really helped was being aware of my body. Whenever I developed niggles or pains I sought treatment straight away by seeing my physio for a tune-up and massage. I highly recommend this (and most health

A bit of advice

Women worry so much about their body and how it looks during pregnancy—but even more so afterwards. And while it's easy to say or think *It doesn't matter what I look like! I grew life!* (which is totally true and absolutely cause for celebration), most women I know do want to get back to their pre-baby bodies. The trick, I think, is to take it easy—on yourself. You *did* create life. You *did* spend nine months renting your body out to a tenant who would never get their bond back in real life. Your body has taken a beating. It will take time to get back to your pre-baby weight and shape. Don't feel bad about wanting to look a certain way, but don't feel bad about not being there yet, either. It'll happen.

funds cover physio treatment, of course). I felt energetic and strong and still had great muscle definition. While I know genetics definitely played a part, I did recover very quickly post-pregnancy and I know that my exercise regime went a long way in making this happen.

With the twins, I really ramped up my pregnancy-safe exercise and Pilates. I knew that I would need to be as strong as I could be to cope with the literal pressure of having two additional people in my body for the foreseeable future, so I made exercise a priority. (Helpfully, lots of people reminded me of this by constantly asking, 'How on earth will you be able to carry twins with your tiny frame?' Always good to add another thing for a pregnant woman to worry about, I reckon!) In the end, despite my slight stature, I carried my twins to 35 weeks (a week longer than the average gestation for identical twins), and in large part, that was down to my fitness program. I did three to four Pilates and prenatal exercise classes a week, plus some light exercise at home on weekends (mainly mat and exercise ball work). I had heard horror stories about women on crutches and wheelchairs in their final trimester with twins and I was determined not to be one of them. Except for the few days around week 28 when I did hobble around on Chris's crutches for a few days, I'm happy to say I wasn't (although by the end I was basically ready to lie down forever and have someone feed me Milo through a tube).

Insta inspo

As with all things social media, there are upsides and downsides to being plugged in while you're pregnant. For me, following mums on Instagram encouraged me to be fit and healthy. In particular, I followed fitness influencer, gym owner, body builder and twin mum Sophie Guidolin (@sophie_guidolin) while pregnant with the twins. She was so strong, fit and healthy—even after her twins—and for me, following her motivated me to stay healthy, too.

That said, other mums can often feel awful when they follow super-fit, super-lean influencers on social media—it leads to unfair comparisons and feelings of resentment, jealousy, sadness or depression. Not good! If you feel like you fit into this category, I'd suggest laying off the social media and spending more time on focusing and looking after *you*. While social media can be great at times and can really motivate people (like me), it can also make people feel awfully shitty about themselves. Look after you and make sure you're using social media in a way that provides a positive outcome. If you're not feeling good about yourself, put the phone away. You just don't need that shit in your life when you're pregnant, or have a beautiful newborn baby to delight in.

Interruption from an expert

Safe exercise during pregnancy

Shira Kramer is an absolute guru when it comes to exercise during pregnancy (and after) and I was so lucky to have had her wisdom and smarts on call during all of my pregnancies and recoveries. Here, I've asked Shira to share some of her best advice, as well as pregnancy workouts you can do at home.

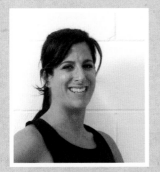

The Women's Health Physiotherapist
Shira Kramer

Why is it so important to stay fit and active during pregnancy (when all you want to do is sit on the couch and eat Maltesers)?

When you fall pregnant, you change in so many ways, both physically and emotionally. And the changes come *fast*. Believe it or not, by week 8 of your pregnancy you are 70 per cent physiologically ready to deliver your baby. Pregnancy should be considered as an Olympic event as the uterus moves from a pelvic organ to an abdominal organ— so we need to train and prepare for this event. Having worked with thousands of pregnant women and new mums over the last decade, I can tell you from firsthand experience that exercise is the key to feeling strong and in control of your body. There are so many things in pregnancy that you cannot control—but if you exercise regularly you can at least control how well you move. We know that regular exercise during pregnancy improves (or maintains) physical fitness, helps with weight management, reduces the risk of gestational diabetes, and enhances psychological wellbeing. We also know that women who exercise during their pregnancy have a faster and smoother recovery after delivery and are better prepared to meet the demands of motherhood.

How do you exercise safely during pregnancy?

Exercising during your pregnancy is essential if you would like to increase your energy levels, minimise aches and pains, keep a healthy weight, maintain muscle tone and control your pelvic floor. However, it is vital to make some modifications to your exercise routine early on in your pregnancy (or even pre-conception) and it can be difficult to know what is safe and where to seek good advice.

There is so much incorrect information out there—whether from well-meaning friends, online research, Instagram posts or outdated books and magazines. If in doubt, please seek advice from your medical consultant or an experienced women's health physiotherapist. Pregnancy is such a fragile time in a woman's life; it's important to be informed by a qualified practitioner so you can make good exercise choices and be kind to your body. In my practice I have seen countless woman who were so enthusiastic to keep fit, but then did the wrong type of training at the wrong intensity.

What are the best exercises to do? And how often should we be exercising while pregnant?

Ideally, we should all be exercising most days of the week, whether we're pregnant or not. Thirty minutes of moderate activity on most or all days of the week—that's the current thinking, and I agree with it. Based on my years of experience of working with mums-to-be, I find that those who prioritise exercise in their daily schedule enjoy the greatest benefits.

Strength and conditioning workouts (like weight training), and core and postural control workouts (such as Clinical Pilates) are great options. Ensure you keep all exercises while pregnant at a moderate intensity and low-impact level. Classes that are pregnancy specific are ideal as they will better meet the demands of your changing body. Working out in groups is also a great way to build social networks with other active mums.

Try to include different forms of exercise in your program, like:

* Strength/resistance training using weights or resistance bands. This will improve (or maintain) muscle tone and strength to better cope with the physical and postural changes of pregnancy and help you prepare for the physical demands of motherhood.

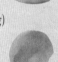

Exercises to avoid during pregnancy

* Contact sports (e.g. hockey, basketball)
* Activities with a high risk of falling (e.g. skiing, horseback riding)
* Scuba diving
* Hot yoga or hot Pilates
* Anything high impact (e.g. running, jumping, high-impact aerobics)
* Heavy weight lifting

Watch out for . . .

* Asymmetrical weight-bearing activities (e.g. wide squats or lunges, or anything standing on one leg)
* Standing still for long periods during exercise—to avoid blood pooling, limit the time you spend standing still and keep your legs moving if you are standing while exercising

Signs it's time to take things down a notch

Exercising during pregnancy should feel good. If you experience vaginal bleeding, regular painful contractions, amniotic fluid leakage or heavy, laboured breathing, stop immediately and see your doctor.

* Low-impact cardiovascular exercise—walking, stationary cycling, swimming, low-impact aerobics.
* Core and pelvic floor exercises—Clinical Pilates is a fabulous way to focus on these areas.
* Relaxation exercises—meditation and exercises that release tension are key to optimising your wellbeing during this time.

What if you don't have much time to spare? What should you prioritise?

First up, there is *always* time to prioritise health and wellbeing. In fact, it should be one of our top priorities all the time! I also firmly believe that, in order to be a good mum, you need to take care of yourself first. However, I do understand that everyone has limits on their time, and some people have more than others. If you don't have a lot of spare time, incorporate as much activity into your everyday life as you can—walking more is a great place to start.

With limited time, I suggest:
* incidental walks (10–20 minutes per day)
* three sets of pelvic floor exercises through the day
* five minutes of core and pelvic floor exercises—while the kettle is boiling, toaster is on, listening to voicemail messages
* integrating short spurts of exercise throughout the day—you do not need to dedicate an hour at a time to get the benefits. Do five minutes of squats, or a session of pelvic tilts while you're watching TV at night. (See Bec's workouts, starting page 98.)

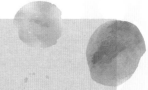

The Borg Scale

Worried about whether you're overdoing it? The Borg Scale is a way to gauge how hard you're pushing yourself, and whether it's safe to do so. It's not so much about your exact heart rate—the scale measures your perception of effort. When you're pregnant, exercising at a *moderate intensity* is considered safe. On the Borg Rating of Perceived Exertion scale, that's a 12 to 14. Basically, aim to get the heart rate up, but still be able to talk. The table below gives you a good indication of what to aim for.

LEVEL OF EXERTION	BORG RATING OF YOUR EXERTION	FOR INSTANCE . . .
None	6	Literally doing nothing. Watching Netflix.
Very, very light	7–8	Putting on make-up
Very light	9–10	Washing dishes, folding clothes
Fairly light	11–12	Walking the kids to school
Somewhat hard	13–14	Brisk walking, sex (!)
Hard	15–16	Bicycling, swimming or other activities that take serious effort. Here, the heart pounds and breathing speeds up.
Very hard	17–18	The highest level of activity you can sustain.
Very, very hard	19–20	A finishing kick in a race or other burst of activity that you can't maintain for long, like a final sprint to the finish line.

Bec's workouts

OK, we're ready to work out! The workouts that follow are the ones that I did during my pregnancies, and I swear by them. They were created by Shira Kramer and they are safe for mamas-to-be. That said, if you have any concerns about starting an exercise program, see your doctor first. This is especially true for women who haven't done much exercise before. In this case, seeing a women's health physio can help.

Remember to . . .

* **Warm up:** Five minutes of gentle stretching before you begin will help loosen up your body and get it ready for activity.
* **And cool down:** Finished? Not yet. Give your body a chance to recover. Go for a gentle five-minute walk to cool down.

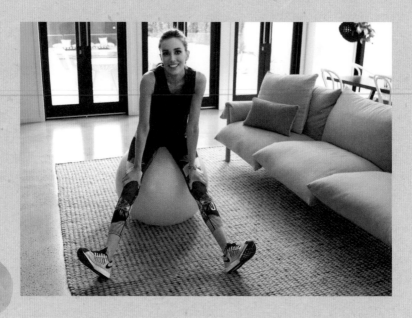

Workout One: Core

Repeat one to five times per week.

MOVE ONE: PELVIC FLOOR MUSCLE EXERCISE

OK, you've heard a lot about the pelvic floor and core over the past few pages . . . but get ready to hear a little more! When you're pregnant, pelvic floor muscle exercises need to be prioritised (and forever after). These muscles control your bowel, bladder and uterus, and they play an important role in controlling where and when you go to the toilet (continence). By exercising your pelvic floor muscles effectively you will be in better shape and much better able to control what goes on down under.

1. Find good posture in any position—sitting, standing, lying on your side or sitting back on your heels.
2. Imagine letting go like you would to pass wind and to pass wee. Let your tummy muscles relax too.
3. Tighten and lift around your back and front passages as if you are holding on to go to the toilet (imagine you're drawing a thickshake up a straw—or lifting your baby up towards your heart).
4. Hold this contraction as you take a breath in and out comfortably.
5. Repeat five times.

MOVE TWO: DEEP ABDOMINAL EXERCISE

The core muscles are the foundations of your body, like bricks in a building. The deep abdominal muscles are important in supporting your back and pelvis. They are often stretched and weakened through pregnancy, which can lead to back pain, poor posture and pelvic floor problems. The outer abdominals can also separate in the centreline (also known as diastasis recti). But by exercising the deep core muscles, your back will cope better with your changing shape and the abdominal muscles are less likely to stretch. This also helps with post-pregnancy recovery.

1. Find good posture in any position—sitting, standing, lying on your side or kneeling on all fours.
2. Imagine letting go like you would to pass wind or to pass wee. Let your tummy muscles relax too.

3. Lift your pelvic floor and then gently and slowly draw in your lower abdominal muscles. Imagine you're giving your baby a gentle hug using your tummy muscles.
4. Hold this contraction as you take a breath in and out comfortably.
5. Hold for one to two breaths and repeat ten times.

MOVE THREE: CORE TO THE WALL—ARM RAISE*

1. Lean your hands (in line with your shoulders) against a wall. Keeping your back and hips straight, and your shoulderblades down, raise one arm up and slowly lower. Keep your elbows soft.
2. Repeat twelve times on each side.

MOVE FOUR: CORE TO THE WALL—LEG RAISE*

1. Lean your hands (in line with your shoulders) against a wall. Keeping your back and hips straight, and your shoulderblades down, raise one leg back behind you, and slowly lower.
2. Repeat twelve times on each side.

MOVE FIVE: CORE TO THE WALL—OPPOSITE RAISES*

1. Lean your hands (in line with your shoulders) against a wall. Keeping your back and hips straight, and your shoulderblades down, raise one arm up and lift the opposite leg back behind you. Slowly lower.
2. Repeat twelve times on each side.

MOVE SIX: SEATED HEEL TAP*

1. Sitting upright with your core engaged, tap one leg forward, and then the other.
2. Repeat twelve times on each side.

MOVE SEVEN: SEATED KNEE LIFT*

1. Sitting upright with your core engaged, lift one knee up, and then the other.
2. Repeat twelve times on each side.

Tip: Make these exercises more difficult by sitting on an exercise ball.

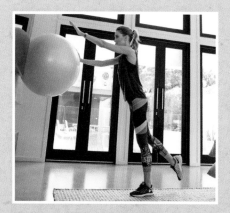

MOVE FIVE Opposite raises

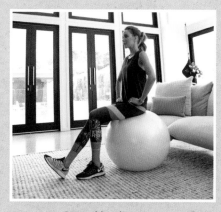

MOVE SIX Seated heel tap

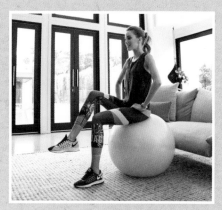

MOVE SEVEN Seated knee lift

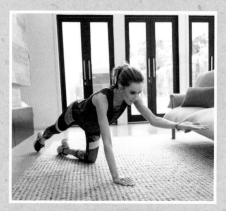

MOVE TEN All fours core—opposites

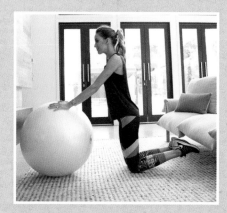

MOVE ELEVEN Roll away

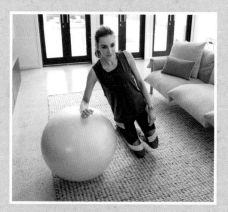

MOVE TWELVE Side lean

MOVE EIGHT: ALL FOURS CORE—ARM RAISE

1. On all fours (with hands positioned in line with the shoulders and knees directly under hips), engage your core and raise one arm forward. Hold for two breaths and slowly lower.
2. Repeat twelve times on each side.

MOVE NINE: ALL FOURS CORE—LEG SLIDE

1. On all fours (with hands positioned in line with the shoulders and knees directly under hips), engage your core and slide one leg back. Hold for two breaths and slowly bring back into place.
2. Repeat twelve times on each side.

MOVE TEN: ALL FOURS CORE—OPPOSITES*

1. On all fours (with hands positioned in line with the shoulders and knees directly under hips), engage your core and raise one arm forward as you slide one leg back. Hold for two breaths and slowly lower.
2. Repeat twelve times on each side.

MOVE ELEVEN: ROLL AWAY*

1. Kneel on the floor with an exercise ball in front of you. Place your hands on the ball and, engaging your core, roll the ball slightly away from you as you lean towards it.
2. Roll the ball back slowly.
3. Repeat twelve times.

MOVE TWELVE: SIDE LEAN*

1. Kneel on the floor with an exercise ball to one side of you (in line with your hip). Leaning your body against the ball, roll the ball slightly away.
2. Roll the ball back using your elbow.
3. Repeat twelve times.

* Tip: As you get better at these exercises, increase the amount of time you hold the positions.

A few tips:

* When you're drawing in your deep abdominal muscles, nothing above the belly button should tighten or tense. Ditto for your legs and butt—if these are contracting, you're not doing the exercises correctly.

* Can't feel your muscles contracting? Change your position (say, from seated to standing) and try again.

* After contracting the abdominal muscles, it's important to relax them. Don't skip this step.

Workout Two: Lower Body Strength

Repeat one to three times per week. Move through this circuit once, have a two- to five-minute break, and then repeat.

MOVE ONE: CALF RAISES

1. Stand tall, with your shoulders back and feet hip-width apart. Raise your heels so you're standing on the balls of your feet.
2. Slowly lower.
3. Repeat fifteen times.

Tip: This is an excellent move for anyone with swollen ankles!

MOVE TWO: SQUATS

1. Stand tall, with your shoulders back and feet hip-width apart. Keep your weight in your heels as you bend your knees and hips (as if you're going to sit on a chair).
2. Slowly come back up.
3. Repeat fifteen times.

MOVE THREE: SQUATS WITH TURN-OUT

1. Stand tall, with your shoulders back and feet hip-width apart and turned out to either side. Keep your weight in your heels as you bend your knees and hips (as if you're going to sit on a chair).
2. Slowly come back up.
3. Repeat fifteen times.

MOVE FOUR: EXERCISE BALL BRIDGE

1. Sit on an exercise ball and walk your feet out until you're almost lying down, and your shoulders are resting on the ball. (Your feet should be in front of your knees.)
2. Slowly raise and then lower your hips, keeping the weight in your heels.
3. Repeat fifteen times.

MOVE FIVE: CLAM

Level One

1. Lie on one side, engage your core, and bend your knees. Keeping your heels together, raise your upper knee. Picture a clam opening.
2. Repeat fifteen times on each side.

Level Two

1. Lie on one side, engage your core, and bend your knees. Hover feet off the floor slightly. Keeping your heels together, raise your upper knee. Picture a clam opening.
2. Repeat fifteen times on each side.

Level Three

1. Lying on one side, engage your core, and bend the knee closest to the floor while straightening the upper leg.
2. Lift upper leg and slowly lower.
3. Repeat fifteen times on each side.

Tip: You should feel these in your buttock muscle and not in your leg—adjust your starting position by moving your knees further forward or back until you feel it in the right spot.

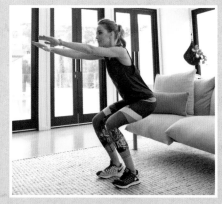

MOVE TWO Squats

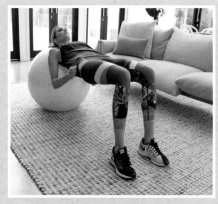

MOVE FOUR Exercise ball bridge, starting position

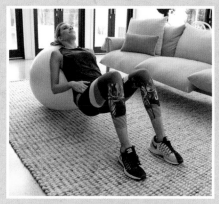

MOVE FOUR Exercise ball bridge, dipped position

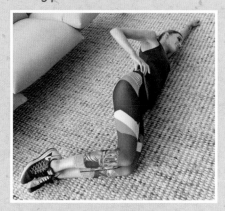

MOVE FIVE Clam, level one

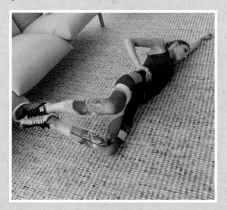

MOVE FIVE Clam, level two

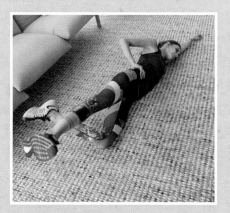

MOVE FIVE Clam, level three

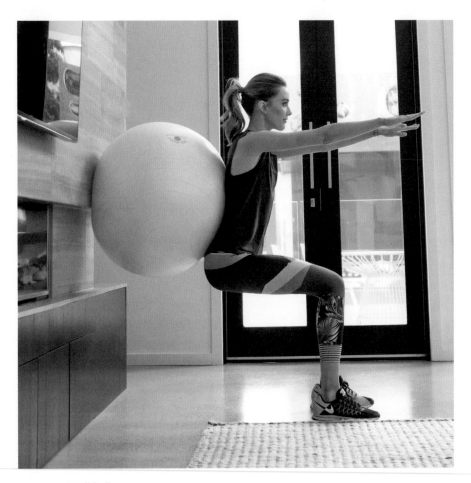

MOVE SIX Wall ball squat

MOVE SIX: WALL BALL SQUAT

1. Prop an exercise ball against a wall and lean into the ball with your lower back.
2. Bend your knees to squat down into a seated position.
3. Slowly stand.
4. Repeat fifteen times.

Tip: This is a great exercise to prepare you for labour! To make it more intense, hold the squat for longer—try for 15 seconds, 30 or even 45!

Workout Three: Upper Body Strength

Repeat one to three times per week. Move through this circuit once, have a two- to five-minute break, and then repeat.

MOVE ONE: **WALL BALL PUSH-UP***

1. Lean an exercise ball against a wall at chest height, and position your hands on the ball.
2. Keeping your back and hips straight, and shoulderblades down, engage your core and slowly lower yourself towards the ball by bending your elbows.
3. Push into the ball to straighten your arms and return to the starting position.
4. Repeat fifteen times.

MOVE TWO: **TRICEP WALL BALL PUSH-UP***

1. Lean an exercise ball against a wall at chest height, and position your hands on the ball, keeping your arms close to your chest and tucked in at the sides.
2. Keeping your back and hips straight, and shoulderblades down, engage your core and slowly lower yourself towards the ball by bending your elbows.
3. Push into the ball to straighten your arms and return to the starting position.
4. Repeat fifteen times.

MOVE THREE: **DIAMOND WALL BALL PUSH-UP***

1. Lean an exercise ball against a wall at chest height, and position your thumb and index fingers on the ball in a diamond shape.
2. Keeping your back and hips straight, and shoulderblades down, engage your core and slowly lower yourself towards the ball by bending your elbows.
3. Push into the ball to straighten your arms and return to the starting position.
4. Repeat fifteen times.

* Tip: These exercises can also be done without an exercise ball.

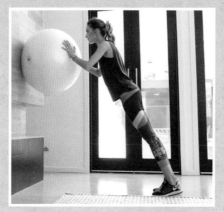

MOVE ONE Wall ball push-up

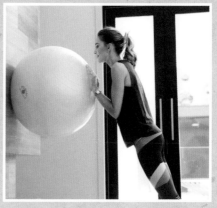

MOVE TWO Tricep wall ball push-up

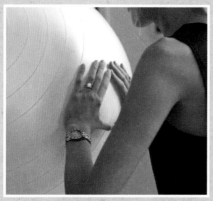

MOVE THREE Diamond wall ball push-up, hand position

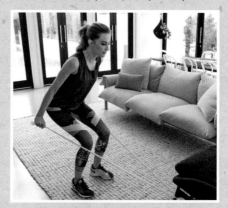

MOVE FOUR Squat and row

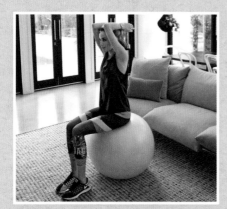

MOVE FIVE Tricep overhead extension

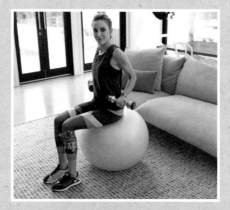

MOVE SIX Upper back pull backs

MOVE FOUR: **SQUAT AND ROW**

1. Standing tall, hold a theraband (resistant elastic bands available from sports stores) in front of you, hooked over something heavy for stability (a table leg, for instance).
2. Squat down by bending knees and hips, and pull your arms back at the same time by squeezing your shoulderblades together.
3. Push your heels into the ground and squeeze your glutes to stand up again.
4. Repeat fifteen times.

MOVE FIVE: **TRICEP OVERHEAD EXTENSION***

1. Sit tall on an exercise ball or chair. Hold a weight (approximately 1–3 kilograms) above your head using both hands.
2. Bend your elbows so the weight lowers down behind you.
3. Slowly extend your arms to bring the weight above your head again.
4. Repeat fifteen times.

MOVE SIX: **UPPER BACK PULL BACKS***

1. Sit tall on an exercise ball or chair and hold a weight (approximately 1–3 kilograms) in each hand, palms facing forward.
2. Reach arms forward, then pull back with elbows at 90 degrees, drawing your shoulderblades together.
3. Repeat fifteen times.

MOVE SEVEN: **SHOULDER RAISES***

1. Sit tall on an exercise ball or chair and hold a weight (approximately 1–3 kilograms) in each hand, with your elbows bent at 90 degrees.
2. Lift your arms sideways until they are in line with your shoulders.
3. Slowly lower.
4. Repeat fifteen times.

* Tip: You can further challenge your core by bringing your feet closer together.

MOVE EIGHT: **BICEP CURLS**

1. Sit tall on an exercise ball or chair and hold a weight (approximately 1–3 kilograms) in each hand, palms facing forward.
2. Slowly bend your elbows, bringing the weights towards your shoulders. Lower slowly.
3. Repeat fifteen times.

Tip: You can also perform this exercise with a theraband. To make it more intense, try lifting one leg off the floor slightly as you bend at the elbows.

MOVE NINE: **SINGLE ARM ROWS**

1. On all fours, with hands positioned beneath the shoulders and knees directly under hips, hold a weight (approximately 1–3 kilograms) in each hand.
2. Engage the core and lift your left arm up and forward.
3. Repeat fifteen times on the left.
4. Repeat fifteen times on the right.

MOVE TEN: **TRICEP KICK BACK**

1. On all fours, with your left hand positioned beneath the shoulders and knees directly under hips, hold a weight (approximately 1–3 kilograms) in your right hand.
2. Move your right hand to your hip with your right elbow bent and close to your body.
3. Straighten your elbow and press the weight towards the ceiling. Bend to lower back down slowly.
4. Repeat fifteen times on the right.
5. Repeat fifteen times on the left.

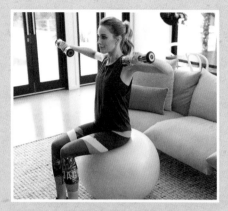

MOVE SEVEN Shoulder raises

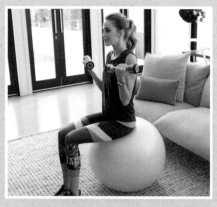

MOVE EIGHT Bicep curls

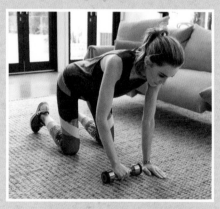

MOVE NINE Single arm rows, starting position

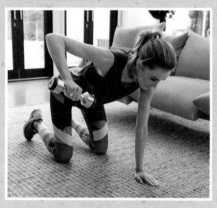

MOVE NINE Single arm rows, second position

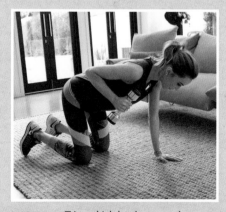

MOVE TEN Tricep kick back, second position

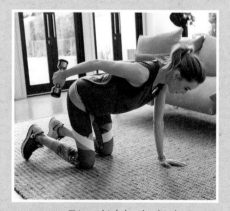

MOVE TEN Tricep kick back, third position

Cool Down Stretches

MOVE ONE: PELVIC CIRCLES
1. Standing tall, or sitting on an exercise ball (or on all fours), move your hips in a smooth, circular motion. Keep your head and shoulders still, and your back straight.
2. Repeat ten times in each direction.

MOVE TWO: SIDE TILT
1. Standing tall, or sitting on an exercise ball (or on all fours), with your head and shoulders still, move your hips from side to side, ensuring your back is straight.
2. Repeat ten times in each direction.

Tip: this is a great stretch to do any time of day, especially when your lower back is aching.

MOVE THREE: PELVIC FORWARD AND BACK TILT
1. Standing tall, or sitting on an exercise ball (or on all fours), with your head and shoulders still, move your hips forward and backwards, keeping your upper back still.
2. Repeat ten times in each direction.

MOVE FOUR: UPRIGHT CHEST STRETCH
1. Standing side-on to a wall, place your hand on the wall at chest height. Turn away from the wall—you should feel a stretch across your chest and shoulder. Hold for 30 seconds.
2. Change sides and repeat.

MOVE FIVE: NECK SIDE STRETCH
1. Sit or stand tall and tilt your head sideways, taking your ear down to your shoulder. Hold for three breaths and stretch to the other side.
2. Repeat three times.

MOVE SIX: NECK CIRCLES
1. Sit or stand tall. Gently roll your neck forward in a half circle.
2. Repeat ten times.
3. Roll in the opposite direction.
4. Repeat ten times.

MOVE SEVEN: SHOULDER ROLLS
1. Sit or stand tall. Roll your shoulders slowly upward, then back down.
2. Repeat ten times.

MOVE EIGHT: CAT STRETCH
1. On all fours, relax your head and allow it to droop.
2. Round your back towards the ceiling. Hold for ten seconds and relax.
3. Repeat three times.

MOVE NINE: CALF STRETCH
1. Stand tall and take one leg behind you. Keeping your back knee straight and toes facing forward, bend the front knee.
2. Hold for 30 seconds.
3. Repeat with the other leg.

MOVE TEN: QUAD STRETCH
1. Lying on your side, bring the foot on top behind you by bending your knee.
2. Holding your ankle gently, pull the foot towards your bum.
3. Hold for 30 seconds.
4. Repeat on the other side.

MOVE ELEVEN: BOOK OPENERS
1. Lying on your side with your knees bent and arms straight in front of you (hands clasped), slowly move your top arm across your body and draw the shoulder down towards the floor, keeping knees together.
2. Hold for 30 seconds.
3. Repeat three times, then swap sides.

weeks 18–21

What's happening with baby

Exciting times—this month, you'll start to feel your baby move! At first it might feel like indigestion, but eventually you'll notice a fluttering sensation. That, my friend, is your baby.

What's happening with you

You're probably still feeling quite tired, but rest assured (sorry, pun intended) that soon you'll feel more energised. In the meantime, enjoy some downtime when you can, and try not to expect too much of yourself.

Size-wise . . .

Your five-month-old baby is now the size of a banana.

Month 5

Pregnancy hormones

Ah, pregnancy hormones. One minute you're on top of the world, staring at your preggo skin and wondering exactly what's made it so glowy and perfect; the next, you're in the foetal position, rocking back and forth, tears streaming down your face.

It's a roller-coaster, that's for sure.

For me, the pregnancy hormones really hit when I had the twins. It was a completely overwhelming time, particularly in the beginning, when I was trying to wrap my head around the idea that I'd have not one, but two newborns to care for. Add to that the risks of carrying twins (especially identical ones), and I was pretty much at breaking point.

When I was fourteen weeks pregnant with the boys, I broke.

Oscar was playing footy inside (I know, I know, totally not allowed—but in my defence, we have no backyard . . . and I was pregnant with twins, taking care of two other small people) as I sat on the couch with a Milo, wondering exactly how I was going to deal with having twins. I was almost finished the Milo, and as I craned my head back to get that last little bit (#nojudgement please), Oscar kicked the ball, smashing the cup into my face.

I broke down in tears.

Pregnancy does weird shit to you, it just does. Poor Oscar was so upset that he had hurt me, but it wasn't even that—it was the fact that I was already entirely on edge, almost waiting for the thing that I knew would tip me over. I cried and cried and cried—one of those massive, never-ending cries that makes your eyes puffy for days afterwards.

But after that, I was OK.

If you're feeling emotional—high, low or somewhere in between—know that this is perfectly normal and reasonable. You are growing a tiny human inside your body. Crazy stuff is happening. You'll be OK eventually, but for now, give yourself a break if you feel a little nutso.

Baby brain: real or just me?

Apparently 'baby brain'—that is, forgetting random stuff when you're pregnant, have just had a baby, or have given birth within the past ten years—is not a real thing. Apparently.

But forget the science (or lack thereof). For me, baby brain was definitely A Thing. When I was pregnant—particularly with the twins—I just could not keep track of anything. I would routinely forget where I'd parked my car. At the airport, I picked up bags that weren't mine. I left Billie at Chris's parents' house and totally forgot I was meant to pick her up. I left an open-flame fire on all day long. One day, Chris came home and thought we'd been broken into—all the doors were wide open. After putting down the kitchen knife and realising that everything was fine, he figured out that it was all me. I'd left without so much as closing the screen door. Oops.

My point is, even if science tells you baby brain isn't real, don't worry if you feel like you're in kindergarten again while you're pregnant. You've got a lot going on. Your brain can only do so much.

Birth classes: Yay or nay?

Before I got pregnant with Oscar, my only knowledge of birth classes came from Hollywood movies. I assumed that, in signing up for prenatal classes, I would be sitting, my legs outstretched, between Chris's legs, his hands on my tummy as we both practised our breathing. *Hoo-hoo ha. Hoo-hoo ha. Hoo-hoo ha.* And so on. For like, the next six weeks.

Except, you know what? Most birth classes do not teach you breathing techniques at all. Is this not the greatest lie we have been fed as women (apart from, of course, 'natural childbirth is the only way to go'—but more on this later)? Most prenatal classes are actually about the logistics of birth: how to spot the signs of labour, when to call (and then go to) the hospital, what your pain relief options are, who will look after you in hospital, who can come into the birthing suite with you, what will happen after your baby is born. In other words, stuff you probably haven't thought much about, but you absolutely need to know.

If you're a first-time parent, I absolutely recommend doing your hospital's prenatal classes. The classes will show you around the hospital (because getting lost mid-contraction isn't exactly ideal), how to tell whether you're in labour (or if you've just wet your pants a bit), what actually happens during labour (yes, there will be videos; yes, they will be graphic; yes, you will see naked vaginas*), and what happens if you need to have intervention, like forceps, a ventouse (a vacuum that assists your baby's delivery) or a caesarean section. Usually hosted by a hospital midwife or doctor, the classes will run you through your pain-relief options (heat packs, gas, epidural; and for caesareans, local and general anaesthetic) and any side-effects you might experience. They'll tell you what to bring in your hospital bag, and what can probably stay at home (spoiler alert: you will *not* have the time or inclination to flatiron your hair). They'll explain birth plans and who you should show yours to (if you have one), and when to come into the hospital when it's go

---

*And probably a *lot* of pubic hair. Every one of these videos seems to have been made in the seventies.

time (some hospitals let you come straight away, others prefer you to wait at home until your contractions are a certain time apart).

They will not, at any point, teach you how to breathe.

Nevertheless, I think birth classes are great for first-time parents. They assuage any fears you might have, you can ask all the questions you want, and there's usually a packet of Arnott's Assorted, too. (Though from experience, I can tell you that the Kingstons are almost always gone before you get there. Bloody midwives.)

What if I do want to learn to breathe?

Besides the classes that hospitals run (which are generally either free or inexpensive), there are also private birth classes that can teach you specific birthing techniques. While I didn't do any of these personally, I'd say go for it if you'd like to approach childbirth with some birthing skills in your arsenal. That said, birth is over pretty quickly (relatively speaking, of course) and I do feel like sometimes we can spend so much time focusing on labour itself that we forget the real challenge: raising a child. To each their own, though—I know plenty of women who have loved their calm birth courses, and if it helps you prepare for childbirth, go for it.

Interruption from an expert

Second trimester ultrasound

Ah, the second trimester ultrasound—this, my friends, is the fun one. Your baby will suddenly look like a real baby. You'll see their little face in profile, their hands and feet kicking, and of course, you'll hear their heartbeat. But the second trimester ultrasound is about more than just warm and fuzzy feelings—so here's Dr Andrew Ngu to explain why we have them.

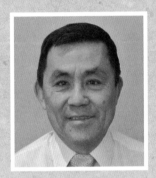

The Ultrasound Expert
Dr Andrew C.C. Ngu

The second trimester ultrasound is the one most parents look forward to from the day they find out they're going to *be* parents—this is the big one. You can find out your baby's sex, see your little one waving about, and get a better sense of who this person inside you really is. But this is also a chance for your medical team to check foetal development and look for any abnormalities. This ultrasound is usually performed at 20–22 weeks.

What does this ultrasound look for?

It assesses foetal development, the amniotic fluid volume, the location of the placenta and the length of the cervix. Your ultrasound technician will measure the head, body and the thighbone to confirm normal growth. They will also check development of the foetal heart and brain. Other things the second trimester ultrasound checks for:

* **The position of the placenta:** You want to make sure the placenta isn't blocking the cervix. If you do have a low-lying placenta, you'll have another ultrasound at 34 weeks to

confirm the position of the placenta. When the placenta continues to be low it may cause bleeding during late in pregnancy.

* **Cervical incompetence**: In this condition, the length of the cervix is shorter than it should be, and is best diagnosed by measuring the length of the cervix by ultrasound. Some women are more prone to cervical incompetence if they had previous cervical laser treatment, cone biopsy treatment to the cervix, or repeated dilation and curette (D&C) of the uterus, and it can occur in women with an abnormally shaped uterus.

* **The sex of your baby**: Many parents choose to find out the sex of their baby at this ultrasound.

What if an abnormality is detected? What happens then?

There are two types of structural abnormalities in the foetus: major and minor. Minor abnormalities are things like skin tags and extra digits—things that aren't present normally, but won't significantly affect your child's life—and major ones that may require medical intervention, as they affect your child's quality of life (and sometimes even their ability to survive). When we find more than one abnormality, we check the rest of the baby's genetic make-up by performing an amniocentesis.

Sadly, some abnormalities are not compatible with life or will have a major impact on the quality of life after the delivery. In these cases, a termination of the pregnancy is an option. If there are multiple abnormalities, a genetic study may be warranted. Sometimes the abnormalities may require delivery at a hospital where immediate care is available. Sometimes we are able to intervene during the pregnancy to prevent further changes. And sometimes, it may be just a case of knowing the problem before delivery so that parents are well prepared.

In the event of an abnormality when a termination is being considered, the parents should consider counselling from specialists like a geneticist, paediatrician, paediatric surgeon, paediatric cardiologist or paediatric neurologist, depending on the nature of the problem.

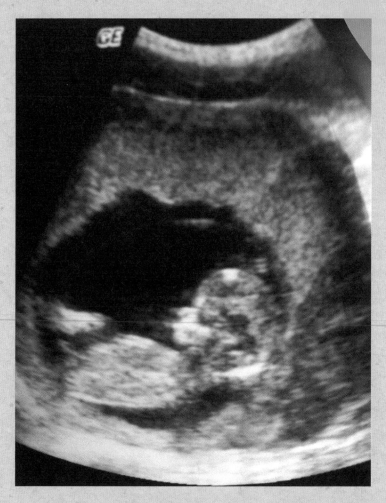

Oscar just sitting back and relaxing. Netflix and chill, anyone?

Eating for two . . . or three

I've always loved to bake. My sister and I would rush home from school every day and make something sweet to feast on before dinner—usually microwave brownies. Throughout all three of my pregnancies I baked and baked and baked . . . and then when I was finally done, I baked a little more. And trust me, I'm not one of those no-sugar, no-dairy, all-vegan raw cookies people. No way. Give me good old-fashioned, old-school baking: slices, biscuits, brownies, cakes—all of it. And give me *all* the sugar, *all* the butter and *all* the good stuff.

Growing twins is a pretty epic event. You're hungry enough growing one baby, but two babies is in a league of its own. To keep up with my insatiable appetite and to make sure I was growing nice, big, healthy babies (size was important as I knew they would come early), it was important I give them the calories they needed. I did this by eating *loads* of baked goods. While I know that it's important to eat well during pregnancy (lots of fresh fruit and veg, wholegrains, dairy and so on), I also think you should indulge yourself and give in to your cravings. What your body is going through is *weird*. It's also hard. You deserve a treat. And you should not feel guilty about it.

With this in mind, I've included my go-to muesli recipe, which is full of healthy nuts, seeds and fats. Lots of women (me!) find they get, ahem, quite blocked up during pregnancy. It's all of the progesterone and relaxin hormones coursing through your body, reducing the 'squeeze' in your smooth muscle, which means your digestive tract becomes quite lax and struggles to push through the poo (welcome to biology, as taught by Rebecca Judd). This muesli is full of fibre, which should keep things moving (drink lots of water and top up with Metamucil, too).

A quick warning—I am so sorry if you have gestational diabetes (poor love). I suggest you quickly flip the recipe pages. It will only leave you salivating and craving these goodies. Completely unfair.

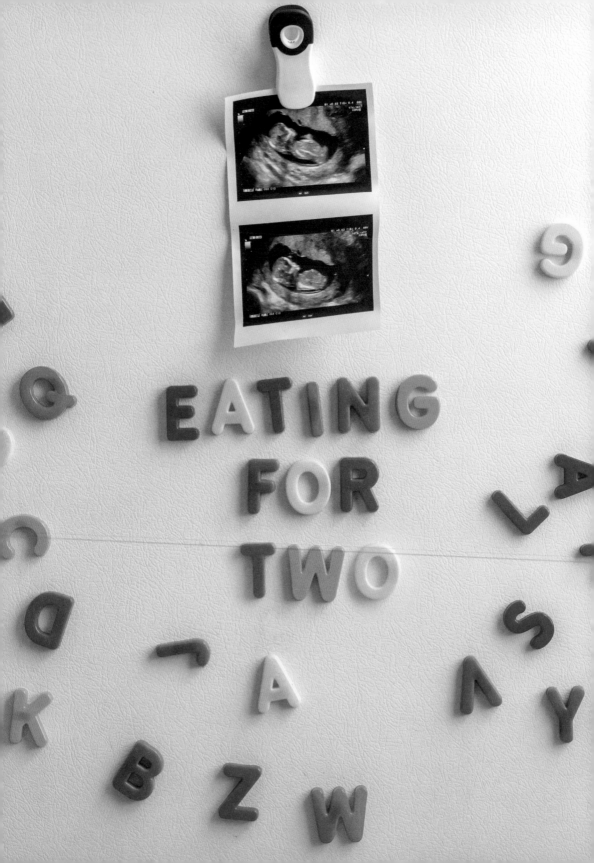

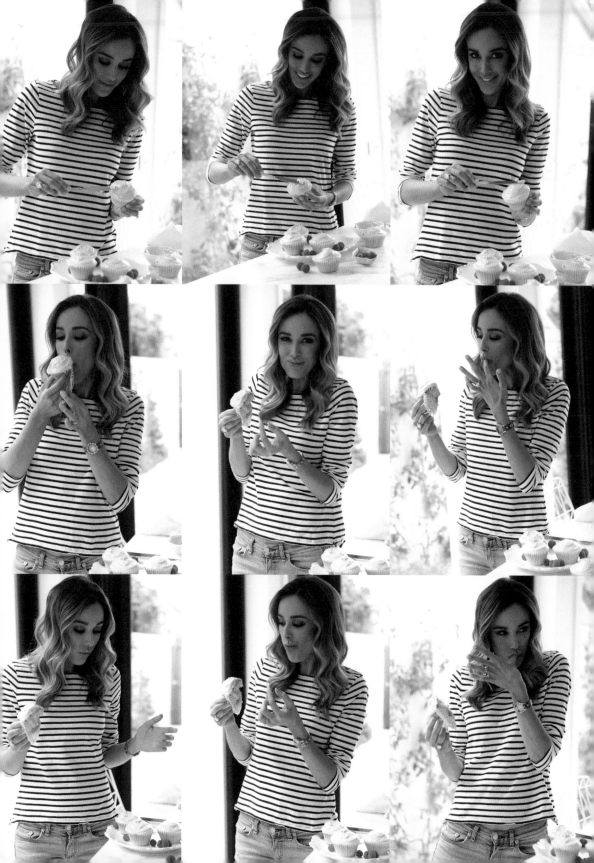

Make-you-go muesli*

I ate this for breakfast daily during most of my pregnancies, with unsweetened Greek yoghurt and fresh berries (when they weren't ten dollars a punnet) or chopped, fresh pear (also a good bowel booster). With the muesli, just add whatever you have at the time. Sometimes I'd swap the pecans for almonds or the pepitas for sunflower kernels. Other times I'd chuck in everything I had. There aren't really any rules—just do whatever floats your boat.

Ingredients

4 cups raw, whole rolled oats
½–1 cup pecans (or whatever nuts you have), chopped
½ cup pepitas
½ cup sunflower kernels
½ cup desiccated coconut
½ cup linseeds (or sometimes I'd use LSA mix—linseeds, sunflower seeds and almonds—instead, added after roasting)
½ cup chia seeds (any type, added after roasting)
4 tablespoons raw honey or maple syrup (or both)

Method

1. Preheat oven to 180 degrees Celsius (fan forced) and grease an extra-large baking tray (you can also do this in batches if your tray or oven isn't big enough).

2. Place all ingredients (minus LSA and chia seeds) onto the baking tray and mix with your hands so everything is evenly spread.

3. Toast in oven for ten minutes. Remove and mix with a spoon, re-spreading the ingredients so the untoasted parts underneath are now on top.

4. Place back in oven for five minutes, remove and mix again. If you think it needs more toasting, place back in oven for another five minutes. Repeat until you have achieved your desired toastiness.

5. Add chia seeds and LSA, allow to completely cool and then store in airtight containers.

6. Serve however you like—with yoghurt or milk, and fresh or dried fruit. When I went out, I would take handfuls of this in Ziploc bags as snacks.

* Cos it makes you go. Get it?

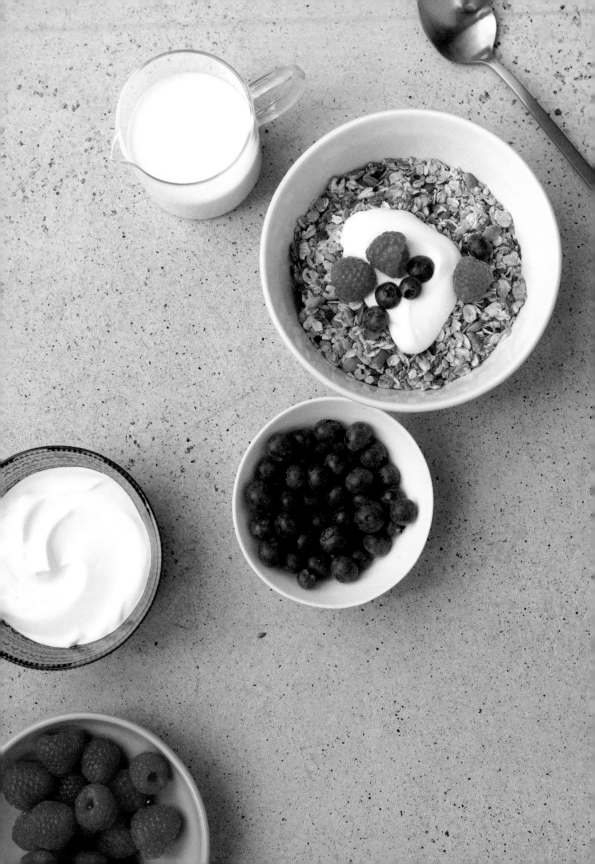

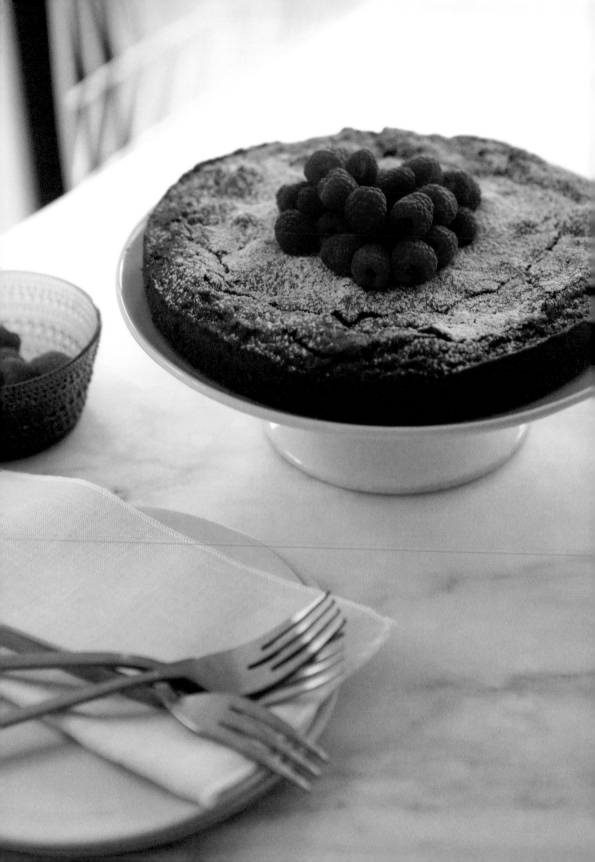

Best-ever gluten-free chocolate cake

I know I said I'm not about no-dairy, no-sugar, blah blah blah . . . but some people genuinely can't tolerate gluten, so this is for them. But this cake is also totally more-ish because it's incredibly dense and moist, due to the almond meal we use in place of flour. It turns out quite flat (because there's no raising agent or flour), but don't let that put you off. It's so bloody good.

Ingredients

200 g almond meal
200 g drinking chocolate
200 g butter (at room temperature)
200 g caster sugar
5 eggs

Method

1. Preheat oven to 160 degrees Celsius (fan forced).

2. Mix all ingredients together in bowl until combined.

3. Bake in 24-centimetre springform tin for 40 minutes.

4. Dust with icing sugar and top with fresh raspberries.

Butter cupcakes with raspberry icing (AKA Billie's pink cupcakes)

Such an easy recipe, which results in the perfect cupcakes: moist, springy, sweet (but not sickly). Billie and I bake these weekly, experimenting with making the perfect pink colour with the raspberries (which provide an all-natural food colouring as well as a bit of zing). Thanks Phillippa Grogan of Phillippa's Bakery in Melbourne for the hot tip. Makes 12.

Ingredients

Cupcakes
250 g soft butter
1 cup caster sugar
3 teaspoons vanilla extract
4 eggs
2 cups self-raising flour, sifted
1 cup milk

Icing
1 ½ cups icing sugar, sifted
25 g soft butter
Half a punnet of raspberries, plus extra for decoration
Milk for desired consistency

Method

1. Preheat oven to 180 degrees Celsius (fan forced).

2. Cream butter and sugar until fluffy using mixer.

3. Add vanilla extract.

4. Add eggs one at a time, whisking well.

5. Add flour and milk a little at a time, alternately.

6. Spoon into cupcake paper cases (I place these in a muffin tray to hold shape) and bake for twenty minutes or until a skewer comes out clean from the middle.

7. Meanwhile, for icing, place icing sugar and butter into a bowl.

8. Squash raspberries in a sieve with the back of a spoon, allowing the juice to drip into bowl with icing sugar and butter.

9. Add small amounts of milk to butter–raspberry mixture. Stir to reach your desired consistency.

10. After allowing cupcakes to completely cool, spread icing over cupcakes and top each with a raspberry.

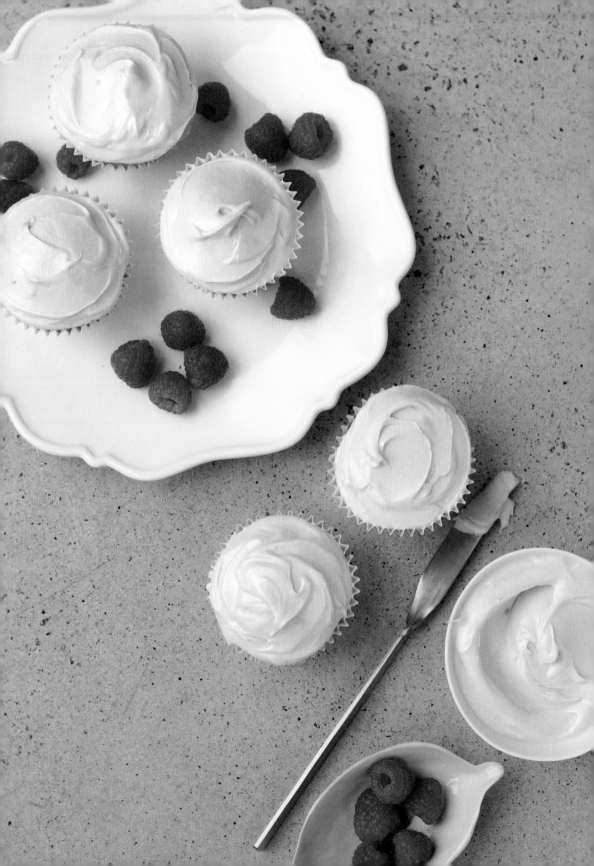

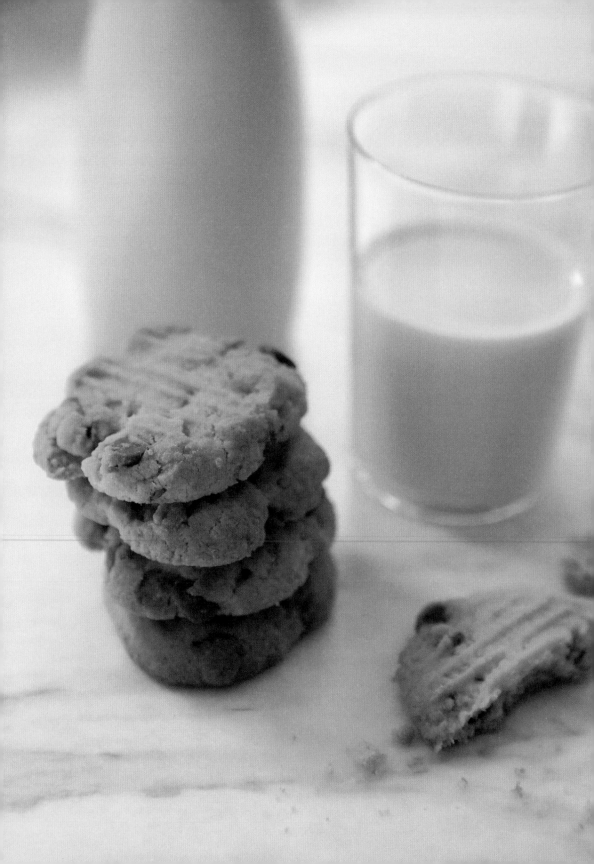

Coconut choc chip cookies

OK, OK—I know everyone says their choc chip cookie recipe is the best ... but believe me, this is the ultimate choc chip cookie! Plus, it's dead easy. What makes it so spesh? Three things: condensed milk, coconut and (of course) a shitload of chocolate. (I usually use milk chocolate but have been known to chuck in some dark and white chocolate chunks, too.) Makes 20.

Ingredients

125 g butter
¼ cup brown sugar
3 tablespoons condensed milk
A few drops of vanilla essence (experiment according to your taste)
¾ cup plain flour
¾ cup desiccated coconut
1 teaspoon baking powder
1 ½ cups chocolate chips

Method

1. Preheat oven to 160 degrees Celsius (fan forced).

2. Cream wet ingredients until light and fluffy.

3. Add dry ingredients and mix together well.

4. Roll into balls and flatten with a fork onto a greased or lined baking tray.

5. Bake for twenty minutes or until golden (keep an eye on them).

Broken biscuit slice

Thanks to my dear friend Jan who made these for me and shared her prize recipe. I would devour the entire tray in one sitting—I dare you not to.

Ingredients

110 g butter
1 ½ tablespoons raw cacao powder (or cocoa)
1–1 ½ tablespoons raw, runny honey
225 g (15) McVitie's Digestive biscuits
Large bar of milk chocolate, for topping

Method

1. Gently melt all ingredients (except biscuits) in a saucepan.

2. Blitz the biscuits to a crumb in a food processor.

3. Add biscuits and wet ingredients and mix together.

4. Lightly butter a shallow 28 x 14 centimetre baking tray and press the mixture into the bottom.

5. Place in fridge to cool and set.

6. Melt the chocolate bar in a glass bowl over a bowl of simmering water.

7. Pour and spread the chocolate over the top of the biscuit layer and put back in fridge to set.

8. Put on elastic-waisted pants and eat.

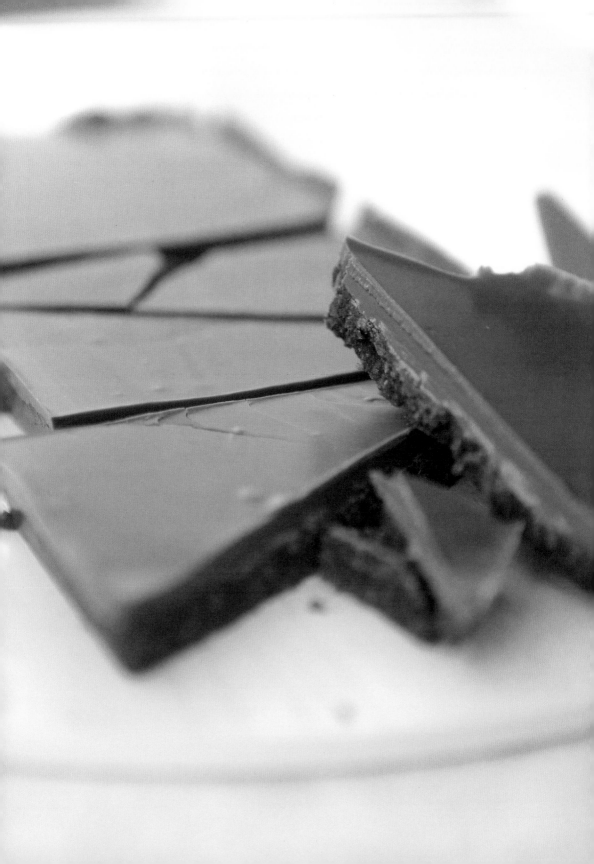

Gross things that are going to happen (sorry)

Pregnancy is beautiful, right? A miracle of nature? An ancient call of womanhood, a sign that we're all sisters?

Um, sure. But it's also, like, completely gross sometimes. Here's a short list of stuff that might happen to your body over the next few months. Enjoy.

* Bloody noses. And not just a small trickle of blood—we're talking blood literally pouring from your nostrils, at all times of the day and night, and completely indiscriminate as to activity (like whether or not you're on live TV. Ahem.) It's thought to be a side-effect of all the extra blood swirling around in your good self.
* Facial hair. Really random, thick, curly hairs growing from weird places, just sprouting up to say hello.
* Acne. Time to break out the Ten-O-Six again.
* Bleeding gums, AKA Bloody Nose's annoying cousin.
* Reflux. Ever eaten a meal, felt totally satisfied and then felt the entire meal want to push itself back up to your mouth? Welcome to reflux!
* Constipation. Not run-of-the-mill, eat-a-prune-and-it'll-be-OK constipation. Oh no. This is akin to losing the ability to push *at all* because it feels like, if you do, you might cause your vag to cave in (AKA prolapse) or push your baby out. Bring a magazine.
* Or, if you're not constipated, maybe you have diarrhoea. Lucky you.
* Constantly wet knickers and funky discharge. Hot tip: bring sanitary pads everywhere you go, as well as an extra pair of knickers.
* Chafing. All that extra fluid down there—not to mention sweat—makes for a lovely environment for chub rub to flourish. Invest in some talc-free powder (like cornstarch) and apply liberally, especially if you're pregnant in summer.
* Pissing your pants. Is that your waters breaking? Nope . . . you just pissed yourself. Watch out for errant wee when you jump, bend your knees too fast, sneeze, laugh, have a Braxton Hicks contraction or don't quite make it to the toilet in time. It's a real thing.

* Varicose veins. They can pop up anywhere, but keep an eye on the backs of your knees and on the outside of your vagina. Sexy, hey?
* Spider veins. These like to spread themselves across your thighs.
* Huge, dark nipples with giant areolas invading your breasts. (Did you ever wonder why you had pink nipples and your mum's were more like a brown colour? Yeah, now you know.)
* DRAM. A Toblerone-like bulge erupting from your tummy where your abs used to be.
* Trouble having sex. Even if you feel up to a dance in the sack, your body might not cooperate. As in, the you-know-what no longer fits in the you-know-where. Coooool.
* Milk leaking out of your boobs!

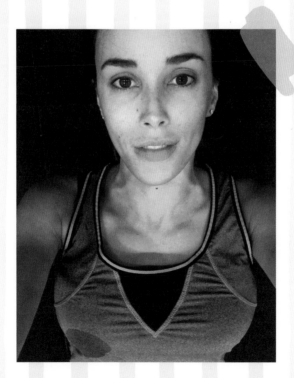

Not the best look!

weeks 22–26

What's happening with baby

At six months, your baby weighs more than your placenta. They'll also start getting into more of a sleep-wake routine, which you might find differs a bit from your own (you're not the only one whose baby kicks furiously at 2 a.m., put it that way).

If your baby was born at 24 weeks, they'd have a good chance of survival as most of their major organs are almost entirely developed. Pretty amazing.

What's happening with you

By now, you probably look preggers—you might find people offering you their seat on the bus and whatnot (and if they don't, it's your right to *insist* that they do). And if you're anything like me, you'll be delirious with hunger.

Size-wise . . .

You've got a baby the size of a sweet potato inside you.

Month 6

Baby gear: What do you really need?

You don't need me to tell you that there is *so much* baby gear out there. There seems to be a product for literally every tiny little problem you or your baby might encounter. Cold wet wipe? You can get a wipe warmer. Baby's hands flailing all over the place when you change them? Yeah, you can buy a wrap to hold their hands in place (I'm not kidding). Can't figure out why your baby is crying? There's a gadget that can tell you. (Wait: no, it can't. This product is ridiculous. But it still exists.)

Anyway, what I'm saying is: there's so much baby stuff out there. Most of it, you don't need. Some of it, you do. Here is a list of the gear I swore by. I hope these products make your life easier, as they did for me.

Newborn essentials

PRAM

OK, you need a pram. But *which* pram? Ask yourself some questions. Where do you live? How often will you use your pram, and in what setting? Do you live in the inner city and plan to visit the supermarket to do your shopping? If so, you will need a big storage basket underneath to cart your purchases back home. Do you plan on exercising with bub in the pram? If so, I'd opt for something with larger, more shock-absorbent wheels. How big is your car? Some prams won't fit in small cars when folded. I encourage you to read all of the reviews about the prams on your wish list prior to purchasing and really find something that's perfect for you and your lifestyle. You'll be using your pram every day, so it's a real investment. Choose the right one and you'll be set. (Oh, and pro tip: always buy the rain cover, even if it's an extra cost. If you don't, you can just about bet that the day you decide to do a 5-k walk it'll start pissing down on you and your baby.)

I chose:

With Oscar, I chose the Stokke Xplory. It was the whizz-bang pram at the time (kind of like the Mansur Gavriel Bucket Bag of prams, if you will), cost a bomb, was perfect for tall people and had a sleek Scandi design which I loved. What I didn't love was the lack of storage. It was such a pain not having a proper basket underneath the pram, as I shopped at the Prahran Market daily and always struggled to cart my groceries home.

With Billie, I had a middle-of-the-road pram in terms of price, design and quality, called the Quinny Yezz. It was fine but not amazing to drive. On the plus side, it had good storage. On the plus-plus side, it was bright pink.

For the twins, I wanted a side-by-side pram that was narrow enough to fit through the skinny doorways of Melbourne cafes but also had great storage, was durable and easy to manoeuvre. The Mountain Buggy Duet was perfect and I love it (it's my favourite of all three of my prams). The only downside? It's so bloody heavy. (Trying to put it in the car after my caesarean was hell. I almost put my back out a few times.) It's also quite large when folded down, so it takes up a lot of space in your car. Still, I'm really happy with it.

COT

Again, there's no getting around the need for a cot. What you choose is up to you—it's a really personal choice. Ensure that your cot meets current Australian safety standards (as well as the mattress you choose) and go from there. My tips are to go for quality and practicality. If you like good design but don't have a huge budget, the cots from IKEA are pretty fab.

I chose:

For Oscar and Billie, I chose an oval cot from Leander. It was beautiful, but oval cots are often smaller and your babies may grow out of them quite quickly, often before they are ready to transition to a big kid bed. They're also hard to find fitted sheets for. But boy, do they look good.

For the twins, I went with the Incy Interiors' Teeny cots, which are sleek and minimal in design with a practical rectangular shape. So much easier to find sheets for.

CAR SEAT

I've always been a fan of the baby capsule that clicks straight onto your pram for easy transitioning without waking baby. I also love the fact that if bub is asleep when you get home, you can just unclick the capsule and bring baby inside easily. My babies transitioned to a rearward-facing car seat (rather than the capsule) around six to seven months (I have tall babies) and then I

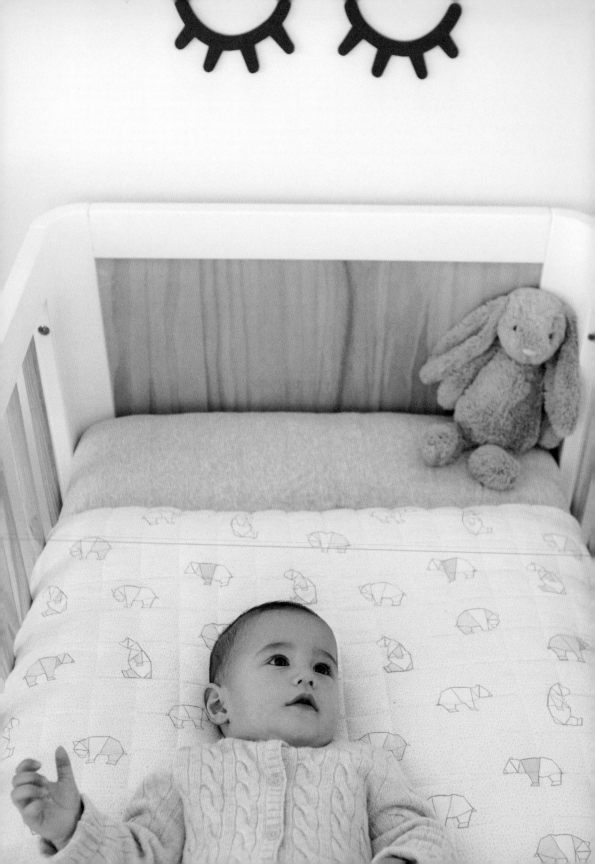

would face it forward once they were tall enough and had good neck and back strength (follow instructions for your bub as every baby—and indeed, car seat—is different).

If you're looking to save some money then you don't need a baby capsule and can go straight into a rearward-facing car seat from the newborn phase (they have newborn inserts) and then face it forward once bub is big enough. This is a far more budget-friendly option.

Always have your car seat installed by a qualified fitter, and ensure you know how to fasten the straps properly. There should be no twists in the straps, and the straps should be tight enough that only one adult finger fits between the strap and the baby. During winter, try not to put bulky clothing on your baby in the car, as this can mess with the straps. Place a blanket snugly over them instead.

My biggest advice when it comes to baby capsules is to do a test run first. Remember when Prince George was born and there was that footage of Prince William trying to get the capsule into the car . . . while literally every photographer in Britain watched? Yeah, I can empathise with Will. When Chris and I were bringing Oscar home from the hospital, we could not for the life of us figure out how to click the capsule into place. We were fumbling around with it for ages, while a carpark full of people stared at us (clearly recognising who we were—so bloody embarrassing). It got to the point where we thought we should just go back into the hospital and stay another night. (OK, not quite that bad, but it was pretty stressful.) In the end, we made an executive decision and swaddled Oscar tightly in a muslin and I held him, with the seatbelt strapped over the two of us, as Chris drove home at a snail's pace (I swear, he didn't go over 20 km/h the entire way home). This was such a rookie error, so I beg of you: test the capsule first.

I chose:
The Maxi-Cosi Mico capsule and Euro car seat.

CHANGE TABLE
A baby change *area* is a must in the nursery, however, a proper change table is something you can go without if you need to. The twins' nursery is upstairs and during the day when they are awake and need a nappy change, I usually

can't be faffed walking upstairs to change them (plus I don't like leaving the other one downstairs by himself). So I keep a spare baby change mattress in a cupboard downstairs with a full supply of nappies and wipes so I can whip it out for a quick change when I need to. I did this for Billie and Oscar too. It's a good idea if you have a multistorey house (or even just a long house) and do your 'living' across different areas.

I chose:
I *love* my BudtzBendix Changing Tower with its Danish design and leather strap. If you're short on space or money you can opt for a change mattress atop your set of drawers. Again, IKEA make great change tables.

For more on change tables, see Styling the nursery, page 152.

SUDOCREM
AKA 'magic cream'. This is the best cream for nappy rash—almost like an instant fix. Even my big kids request 'magic cream' when they've scraped their knees or grazed their shins.

NAPPIES AND WIPES
Another non-negotiable. I've tried them all—literally—and still I have not found the 'perfect' nappy. Again, this will be a process of trial and error. Find the nappies that fit your baby best (i.e. that don't leak) and aren't too harmful to the environment. If you can find a nappy that ticks both boxes, please let me know. As for wipes, I prefer those that don't contain any crap: so no parabens, no fragrance, no sodium lauryl sulfate (SLS) and so on. There are plenty out there that fit the bill.

You can also, of course, buy cloth nappies. I didn't do this, but it's a great way to help the environment and cut down on costs. Don't worry—cloth nappies have come a long way since those terry towelling squares from the eighties. These days, modern cloth nappies have water-resistant covers, leak-proof elasticised leg holes, absorbent padding and a liner. Have a look on Etsy—there are some really cute designs out there. Cloth nappies are a bit more work, and not as convenient as disposables, but using a method called 'dry pailing' is said to make cleaning pretty easy.

NAPPY BAGS

Keep a stash of these near your change table. I know there are those bins that are supposedly hygienic . . . but they just seem like toxic waste containers to me. Even better, if you have plastic grocery bags, give them one more use by chucking dirty nappies in them.

NURSING CHAIR

This is a must-have for late-night feeds (yes, there'll be a few of them). Choose one with a high back and armrests so you can lean back and relax and save yourself weekly visits to the chiro. If you want to stretch out, choose a chair with a matching ottoman or footstool. You're going to be nursing a lot—you may as well be comfy.

I chose:

The Rocking Chair from Adairs, and it's perfect.

FEEDING PILLOW

This crescent-shaped pillow is not only a must-have for breastfeeding (and actually, bottle-feeding) your bub, as it is the ultimate neck and back saver, but it also makes the best preggo belly support pillow when you're heavily pregnant and you're just so darn uncomfortable when trying to sleep. You know that feeling when you're lying on your side and you feel like your belly might just tear off your body from the pressure? Yep, me too. While on your side, wedge this pillow under your bump and down between your knees. Go to sleep. Wake up feeling like you've actually had a rest. Amazing.

BABY CARRIER

As well as a pram, you'll probably also want an infant carrier—i.e. a pack that allows you to strap your baby to your chest or back. Prams are fantastic but if you need to pop out quickly, or do something with an older child, carriers are fantastic. They're also useful when you need to get things done around the house and your baby won't sleep (fun times for all). I swear by them when we go travelling, too. They're also great for dads to wear—they help father–baby bonding.

I chose:
The BabyBjörn Infant Carrier. I've tried a lot of infant carriers but I always come back to the BabyBjörn. They have so many styles to choose from at varying prices but they all have a very similar shape, style and functionality. I find them very easy to use and so comfortable.

BATH
Even if you have a bath in your bathroom, you'll need a baby bath for the first few months. A big plastic tub—nothing fancy—will suffice, as well as good bench space near a tap. We still bathe Tom and Darcy on our kitchen bench. Always use a bath wash with all natural ingredients and without SLS.

BOUNCER
At some point, you will need to put your baby down while you do other things, like pour yourself a glass of shiraz, or reach for the packet of chips you stupidly put in a really high cupboard ages ago. I'm talking here about the sitting kind of bouncer, not the ones you strap to doorways where your baby stands and bounces (to me, they seem quite dangerous). I used to put my babies in their bouncers while I had a shower: I shower, baby watches and bounces away. Everyone's happy and safe, and I get to condition my hair. Win–win!

PORTABLE CHANGE MAT AND WIPES WALLET
There are so many nifty little nappy wallets you can buy these days. They roll out to be change mats (imperative for when you're out and about), and can store a couple of nappies and a slimline wipes packet. Make sure yours can be wiped down and is machine-washable. Check Etsy for some cool designs.

BOOKS
As a speech pathologist I know the importance of reading to your children from a very young age. Did you know that acquiring early literacy skills leads to a higher IQ? I know it can seem silly to read to a newborn—who can't even understand what you're saying—but in fact, constant exposure to language including speech sounds, semantics and syntax all stimulates the language

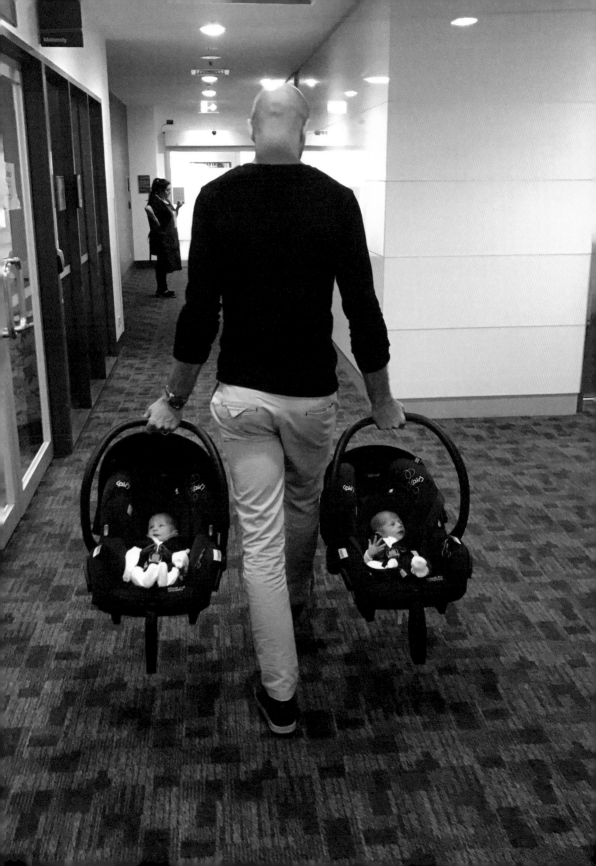

centres of the brain—even in young babies. You'll be amazed at how early exposure to language kicks these centres into gear a lot sooner and helps them to run more efficiently once your baby gets a little older and starts to understand more. So bombard your baby with stories. The more speech sounds and colourful language (ahem, not the naughty type), the better.

My favourites:
I could name hundreds of books here, but my top five for newborns are:
* *Where is the Green Sheep?* by Mem Fox
* *The Very Hungry Caterpillar* by Eric Carle
* *Ten Little Fingers and Ten Little Toes* by Mem Fox
* *Five Little Monkeys* by Eileen Christelow
* *Guess How Much I Love You* by Sam McBratney.

Newborn optionals

TRAVEL COT
You don't need a travel cot, but if you're planning on going anywhere with your little one, you will need to consider buying one. (You can also hire travel cots, or see if your accommodation provides them—more on this in Travel with a newborn, page 288.)
I chose:
The BabyBjörn Travel Cot. This is the Rolls-Royce of travel cots, which means it's amazing, but it's also pretty exxy. I've tried a few travel cots and this is by far the lightest and easiest to erect and dismantle. (If you don't want to get a divorce over a travel cot, I recommend you buy it immediately.) The mattress is also thicker and more comfortable than some of the paper-thin competitor products.

STERILISER
If you're bottle-feeding or using dummies, you'll need a steriliser.
I chose:
I bought the Avent steriliser when Oscar was a baby, and I use it to this day.

BOTTLES

Again, if you're bottle-feeding, you're going to need . . . bottles! However, not all bottles are created equal. There are so many on the market, and the choice can be overwhelming—wide neck, slow flow, peristaltic . . . it doesn't really make sense until you have the baby. Generally speaking, newborns prefer slow-flow nipples with wide necks. Sometimes it's a matter of trial and error, though, so I wish you the best of luck. You'll need about six bottles per baby.

I chose:

On advice from a midwife because my twins were premature, I chose Avent wide neck bottles (which I also used for Oscar and Billie) but paired them with a Pigeon SofTouch Peristaltic wide neck teat. They were perfect.

DUMMY

OK, so everyone and their mother has an opinion on dummies, but personally, I love them. In the early days, I used them to settle my babies to sleep and to encourage them to sleep longer than one 40-minute cycle. (That said, I knew I didn't want my kids to rely on dummies to fall asleep, so I gently weaned them off at about ten weeks, when they were quite happy to let me have them—any later than this and I think it gets tricky.)

I chose:

Natural Rubber Soothers.

BABY BAG (OR JUST A BIG HANDBAG)

Many first-time mums buy a massive nappy bag thinking they'll use it all the time. (Yep, I did this, too.) But honestly, I prefer to use my giant handbag, and then just add a nappy wallet and bottle bag to it, rather than changing bags all the time (or carrying two bags—absolutely not). I cannot fathom how some women wrangle a child (or two), holding their own handbag and another nappy bag. Talk about nightmare. My advice? Choose a big, roomy handbag with lots of pockets (or just buy an organiser that you insert) that can be wiped down.

I chose:

For flights, I take a dedicated nappy bag. I chose a black Country Road bag.

MUSLIN WRAPS/SWADDLES/BUNNY RUGS

I wrapped all of my kids until they were about three months old. Swaddling mimics the cosy nature of the womb, and it also helps babies to stay asleep as they can't move their hands and wake themselves up. For a fail-safe technique, google 'Midwife Cath's Wrap' for a video that shows exactly how to wrap your bub.

SLEEPING BAG

As well as a swaddle, you might want to get a sleeping bag, particularly for the colder months. After wrapping my babies, I would then zip them into a sleeping bag to provide extra warmth. Sleeping bags are better than blankets as they can't be kicked off and can't cover your baby's face.

I chose:

The ErgoCocoon. These come in different fabric weights, so you can choose one that is suitable for the temperature at the time. I used these for my kids from birth until they were about two years old.

THERMOMETER

The only thing more terrifying than cutting your newborn's nails is not knowing what's going on with your baby when they're crying, fussy or won't go to sleep as they normally would. Having a thermometer is so handy for checking whether they are upset because they're sick. Choose a digital thermometer that can take their temp from their forehead (babies *hate* having things stuck in their ears or mouths), and look for one with an in-built light, if you can (useful for night-time).

BLACKOUT BLINDS

This seems OTT until you are desperate for your baby to sleep and will do anything to facilitate that. I know people say that babies can sleep 'anywhere', but after a few months, babies become a lot more sensitive to sounds and light. To block out sun during the day (and the early morning), invest in some blackout blinds. The Gro Anywhere Blind is a portable blackout blind that uses suction caps to attach to windows. They are fab.

Newborn clothing

ONESIES

Forget the fancy stuff, give me a Bonds Wondersuit any day of the week. I was that first-time mum who bought all the cute (and extremely impractical) outfits for poor little Oscar. Within days I figured out that, a) I didn't have time to dress him like a baby sailor every day, and b) babies look just as cute in onesies as they do in miniature tuxedos. Look for suits with zips—so much easier to put on than those with snap buttons.

I chose:

Bonds Wondersuits. Approximately 10,000 of them. (Trust me, you'll need quite a few. Between leaky nappies, cheeky little milk chucks and never-ending dribble, you'll go through a lot.)

BIBS

About 30 should do it. Nope, not kidding. You'll be astounded at how messy and leaky feeding can be—whether you're breastfeeding or bottle-feeding. (And just wait until you get to solids!)

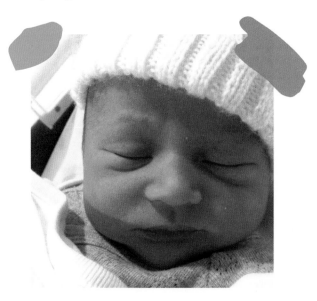

My little one-day-old Oscar. What a dude!

Styling the nursery

When I saw those two blue lines on the wee stick, one of my first thoughts was: baby nursery. With all my kids, I was so excited to style their rooms and create a space that was perfect for them. Styling a nursery is definitely on the 'fun' end of the pregnancy spectrum (at the other end, you'll find extreme sweating and thigh chafing)—the trick is to find a balance between styling for your baby and yourselves. You want the room to be kid-friendly, of course, but you also want it to be stylish and fit in with the aesthetic of the rest of your house. (In other words, no primary colours or Disney characters.)

So, where do you start?

The furniture

First: think about what you really need. You'll need a cot (obvs), some kind of change area (whether that be atop a chest of drawers or a proper change table), a nursing chair for night feeds (and a side table to put your bits and bobs when feeding, like bottles, phone, medication, spare wipes etc.) and lighting. These are the essentials.

Then have a think about anything else you might need to invest in before bub arrives, like extra storage. If your room already has built-in cupboards then you might not need a set of drawers or a new wardrobe. And think about hybrid products, too—some chests of drawers can accommodate a change table on top, saving you a heap of space.

Measure the room and decide where you'll place your furniture. Try to keep the cot away from power points and windows if possible, for safety reasons (electrical outlets can be fire hazards and blind cords are a massive choking hazard).

The hero wall

After you've got the non-negotiables sorted, think about how you'd like the nursery to look—AKA, the fun bit. I like to start with my hero wall and work back from that. Your hero wall is often the wall your cot sits against, or the wall where your nursing chair is positioned. Anchor this wall with artwork—a painting, a print, a photo, a wall-hanging, even a stuffed toy animal head! You could also consider painting this wall with a solid colour or using wallpaper, or even panelling. It looks so schmick.

The vignette

Create a 'vignette' (AKA, a little area of gorgeousness) around your hero artwork where you will style your main pieces of furniture (the cot or nursing chair). Next, add decorative items to your vignette. Think decals, garlands, mobiles, lighting, shelves, beautiful stuffed toys, roof installations. I love stringing garlands across artwork to add a little more interest. The main rule is to have fun with it—and that there are no rules.

Choosing your colours

OK, I lied. There is one rule—choose complementary colours. After you've got your artwork, choose one hero colour from the piece (ideally not the most obvious one) and use this in other decorative items around the room. So if your artwork is a crocheted wall-hanging in peach, grey and white, you might choose to have your other decorative objects in shades of grey. The decorative items will bring the room together in a cohesive way, without looking too contrived. In Billie's nursery, for example, there's gold in the artwork, which has become my hero colour. You might not immediately see all the gold in her room (which is the point—it's meant to be subtle) but it's there—the gold love-heart vase on the wall, the gold triangle on the bedding, the gold fleck in her rug, the gold feet on her rocking horse. Ta-da!

What colour palette is right for you? For girls, I love whites, creams, pale pink, lilac and grey. Throw in a hint of the softest mint and you have the perfect palette. For boys, I love white, grey, black, seafoam green and duck egg blue. A hint of navy looks great, too.

Waiting to find out your baby's sex, but still want to prepare? Go for a safe palette—grey and white with hints of metallic gold and spearmint. Once bub comes, you can go mad buying accessories with colour. You have my permission. The bottom line: you just can't go wrong with a neutral canvas.

The nursing chair

Even if your nursing chair isn't placed against your hero wall, it's still a focal point of the room, so give it a little personality. Place a rug underneath it to anchor it. Add a huge chunky knit, like I did in Tom and Darcy's nursery—not only does it look gorgeous, it's also very useful for late-night, post-feed winter cuddles. A side table with a stack of toys and books is another option.

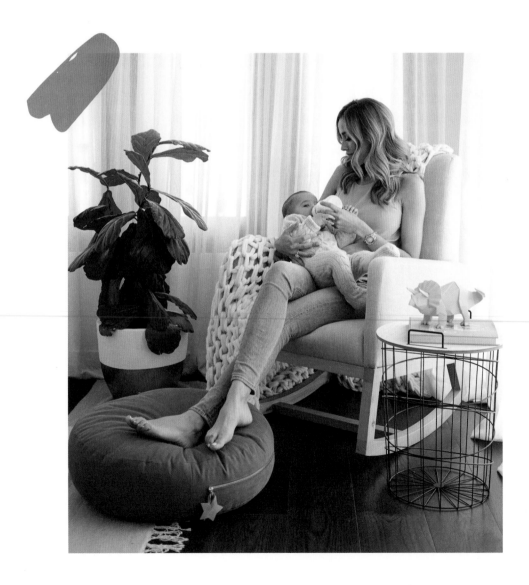

The cot

Which cot? With Oscar and Billie, I went all out and bought a curved Leander cot. It was beautiful to look at, made with impeccable Danish design . . . and cost about as much as a week-long trip to Hamilton Island. While I love a curved cot, I found it harder to find bed linen to fit, and I find they are often a little smaller (a problem when you've married a footballer). If you have long babies like me, they can outgrow them more quickly than a standard rectangular cot. So for the twins I chose the rectangular Teeny cots by Incy Interiors. I love them—zero complaints. For great design at a fraction of the price, IKEA cots are hard to beat.

Lettering

Say it with writing. Think of adding a huge letter (like your child's first initial) or play with wire letters to spell their name out entirely.

Shelving

Shelves serve both a functional and aesthetic purpose. They are a great way to display your bub's treasured items, and you can have fun styling them up so that they become a cute focal point in the room. I love playing around with books, toys and dolls to create little vignettes that take the eye on a journey. Play with shapes and vary the heights. Cluster cute things together—wooden ornaments, blocks or little babushka dolls. Add a light or a hanging garland. Stick to neutral shades mixed in with your hero colours.

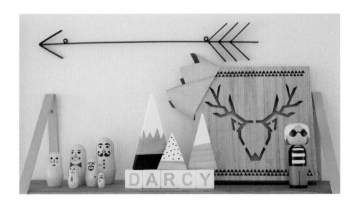

Rugs

Rugs are great for adding softness and warmth to a room. They can also become a focal point if you play with shape, texture or colour. In Billie's room, for example, we used an irregular-shaped cowhide—not something you'd usually find in a kid's room, but it gave the space a relaxed feeling, and stopped it from looking too cookie-cutter perfect. With the twins, I used the colours in their rug as the room's hero colour. See how the tones on the shelf's decorative objects tie back with the colours in the rug? Plus, the fringing gives it a little extra charm.

The bedding

For bedding, neutrals are always best. You can then add a hint of pastel colour or metallic, or bolder colours with accessories like cushions and toys (but be sure to remove these for bedtime). Soft linens and quilted jersey work well for comfort. Because little ones seem to kick off their covers every ten seconds, my kids have always slept in sleeping bags with a blanket or quilt cover over the top, tightly tucked in (see Safe sleeping tips, page 283).

The lighting

One must-have item for every nursery is some form of soft lighting for night feeds and nappy changes. For all of my babies I used a floor lamp which emitted a soft light for late-night shenanigans. I'm also partial to a cute night-light. You can find these in an array of gorgeous forms, from toadstools and dinosaurs to fruit and clouds.

Cushions

Cushions are fab for adding interest. You can pretty much find any shape, style and colour these days, and they're quite affordable. Start with a couple of standard-shaped, textured cushions and then add a character or themed cushion for interest and charm. Think ice creams, clouds, doughnuts, arrows, animal heads, lightning bolts—whatever you want. Have fun!

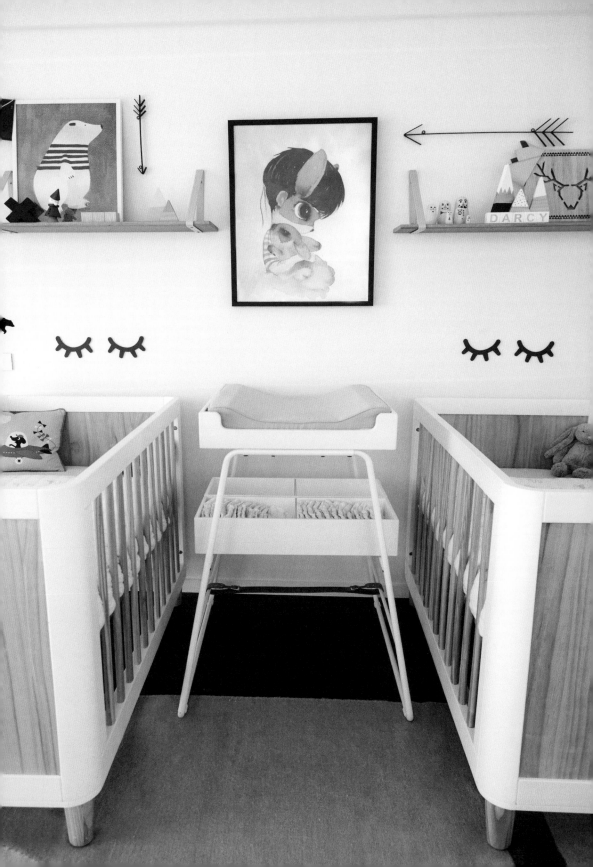

Bec's fave interiors Instas

@adairs The best bedding plus gorgeous quilt covers and coverlets, and the cutest kids' furniture and toys.

@designstuff_group Scandinavian nursery furniture (including the coolest change table ever).

@etsyau Where you will find whatever you're into—they have literally *everything* and are really affordable.

@goldfrankincensemyrrh Feather crowns, dolls, storage houses and accessories (AKA Billie's dream).

@theincystore Great for furniture.

@invitemeshop Decorative objects, hanging garlands, party gear—all super bloody cute.

@jackandjillboxes Personalised boxes (these make great gifts).

@kmartaus Ridiculously awesome and cheap wares for the nursery. Think lighting, rugs, side tables and decorative objects.

@leoandbella A huge selection—bedding, beanbags, books, rugs, night-lights, posters, wall decor, shelves, wallpaper, toys . . . the list goes on. You could pretty much deck out your whole nursery here.

@littleconnoisseur Personalised decor such as floor cushions, bags and key rings.

@littlelibertyrooms An interior decorator with seriously great style.

@miannandco Kids' furniture, lighting, mobiles, wall art, wall hooks, rugs and beanbags.

@mooi_baby Beautiful play mats and bedding.

@norsuinteriors Nordic art and homewares. Great prints and a large selection of frames and hanging options.

@oh.eight.oh.nine A Perth-based interiors stylist and blogger with great style who *always* shares her much coveted supplier lists. This girl is one of my faves.

@petiteinteriorco Beautiful inspo from the world's largest children's interior design studio.

@pretty.in.pine Handpainted, quirky shelves, cupboards and decor (like those cute sleepy eye hangings). This stuff is seriously pretty and full of charm.

@simple.form Scandinavian, Japanese and minimalist design. Great for knick-knacks for your shelves.

@talointeriors Parisian, Scandinavian and Australian decor for babies and kids.

@thelittleinterior Cute kids' decor and knick-knacks.

@winterandvine Wooden swings and shelving that are too cute for words.

@_zilvi Adorable wooden decor.

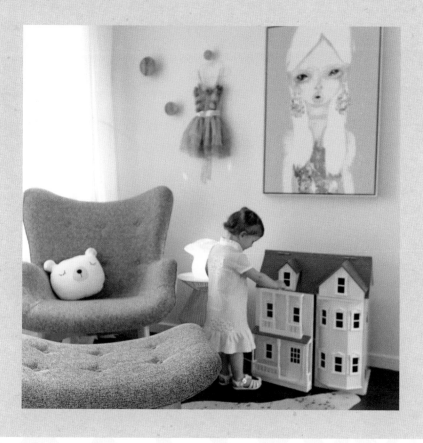

weeks 27–30

What's happening with baby

Your baby is in full-on baby mode. It can hiccup. It can *wee*. The lungs, brain and digestive system are fully formed, but not entirely mature yet.

You've probably noticed that your baby is getting pretty active—from now until the end of your pregnancy, it will be moving vigorously, whether you like it or not!

What's happening with you

If you're finding it hard to keep your Weet-Bix down, you're not alone: heartburn and indigestion are really common at this stage of your pregnancy. I suggest small snacks, often.

You might also have swollen hands and feet, owing to our friend, Water Retention. Try to drink as much water as you can to eliminate this, but also know that post-birth, it does all go away.

Size-wise . . .

We're at the cauliflower stage. Yep. There's a baby the size of a cauliflower all up and in you. Crazy, isn't it?

Month 7

Babymoon time

A lot of people ask me if it's worth it to go on a babymoon. My answer is always (and without fail): *yes absolutely go, are you joking, get out of here right now, go go go.*

So yeah, I'm a big fan of the babymoon.

If you can afford it—and if you can take the time off work—I think you should definitely treat yourself to a babymoon. Having a baby—being pregnant, delivering that baby and then taking care of it for, you know, the next eighteen years—is *hard*. Physically, it's demanding. Emotionally, it's exhausting. And if you thought your days of manual labour ended when you stopped working at Macca's in high school . . . prepare to start all over again. I remember about six weeks after Oscar was born, I was changing his nappy one day and realised, *Oh shit. This is never going to end. I am going to be changing his nappy seven times a day—on a good day—for the next two years.*

So yeah, go on the babymoon.

My babymoons

You don't have to do anything too fancy for your babymoon. I know couples who have gone to Europe, or done a big road trip through America, or even just stayed at home, but personally, I think all you need is a bit of sun (if that's your thing), a stack of books, good coffee (you can have one or two a day, and you may as well have the best you can find), and the willingness to turn your phone and laptop off the entire time.

When I was pregnant with Oscar, I went to Broome with my mum, sister and a friend. (Chris was playing footy and missed out—sorry, babe.) Our girls' trip consisted of sitting on the beach, eating pizza (with ice cream chasers) and watching chick flicks at night. It was the best.

With Billie, we went to Noosa. (Chris even got to come this time.) We swam, drank cocktails (well, mocktails for me), ate indulgent dinners (and plenty of ice cream), slept in and just switched ourselves off from the world. The second time around, it felt even more important to take some time out, because we already had Oscar and it was so nice to have some time that was just for me and Chris.

With the twins, I couldn't fly past 20 weeks. We went further north because it was the middle of winter. We didn't want to go to Noosa (too cold) or fly to Broome (too far), so we settled on beautiful Palm Cove. The weather was perfect every day, and my poor preggo tum got to enjoy some sunshine instead of Melbourne drizzle. (You can take the girl out of Perth, but you can't take Perth out of the girl.)

The babymoon checklist

* Switch off your work email.
* Do not take your laptop. I mean it.
* Book a pregnancy massage. At least one.
* Go out for a special dinner. I will not tell anyone if you decide to have one cheeky glass of wine.
* Read. Take that stack of books that's been sitting on your bedside table and for the love of J.K. Rowling, *read them*. Ditto all those magazines that have been piling up in your living room.

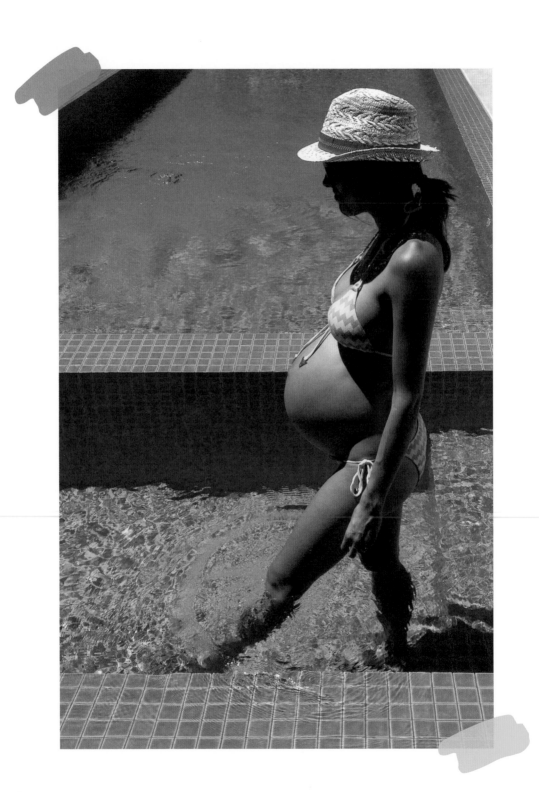

The babymoon staycation

As well as heading to Palm Cove before the twins arrived, we had a little staycation in Melbourne with the kids. If you have a complicated pregnancy, are carrying multiples or have left it a little too late to fly, I highly recommend a staycation. Just not the one we went on.

I thought I was being so clever. It was Oscar's birthday, but I just could not handle the idea of a birthday party. All that setting up and organising and people in my house and cleaning up . . . nope. I couldn't do it. So I asked Oscar if, instead, he'd like to take a few friends to Crown for the weekend. I mean, there's a pool, there's a cinema—it's a kid's paradise! He jumped at the offer and we were set.

Except we weren't. Because just as his friends' parents began dropping their kids off at the hotel, I came down with the worst gastro of my life (you know that scene in *Bridesmaids*? Yeah, that scene. That was me). I said to Chris, 'You're on your own, buddy. Have fun with these five-year-olds.' And off I went to the bathroom in our room at the Crown, where I stayed for the next two days, vomiting, having diarrhoea and wetting my pants (because every time I vomited and my stomach muscles contracted, I would lose control of my bladder). At one point Chris came in to ask if I wanted a cup of tea. I was sitting in a pool of my own wee and couldn't give him a stare that was quite dirty enough. I think he got the hint, though.

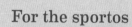

For the sportos

If you're into horse riding or scuba diving, first of all: that is great. I am not, but I salute your commitment to being adventurous and amazing. Second, don't do these things on your babymoon. They're not safe for your bub (or you) and most travel insurance will not cover these activities. (Just tide yourself over by imagining how cute your baby is going to look in jodhpurs in eighteen months' time.)

Before you go

Check the Australian Government's Smart Traveller website for information about the safety of countries you'd like to visit. Regarding airplane travel, consider where you're going when it comes to how far along you are. Babies born in Australia from 28 weeks have a great chance of survival, but if you're going to a country like Fiji or Bali, where the hospital systems aren't always up to our standards, you might want to come back earlier. Always make sure you have travel insurance that covers pregnancy, and if your pregnancy is complicated (for example, multiples) you may want to consider not travelling at all. If you're travelling after 30 weeks, many airlines request a letter from your doctor, confirming you're OK to fly—make sure you've arranged this before you get to the airport.

I suggest heading off before 30 weeks, if you can. This way, you won't be so big that you can't swim, walk around and enjoy yourself, and you'll also be able to fly to most places.

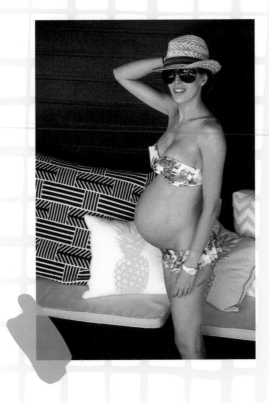

Interruption from an expert

Airline travel

Dr Len Kliman weighs in on travel during pregnancy.

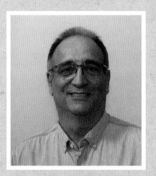

The Obstetrician
Dr Len Kliman

What are the main things to consider when planning travel while pregnant?

Check to see if the country you're heading to is prone to the Zika virus or malaria. The Australian Government's Smart Traveller website will have info on this.

For overseas trips, go before week 30. For interstate, you can fly up to week 34.

Always avoid countries without a good healthcare system, especially after the first trimester, as obstetric care will be less than adequate if you have complications.

What are the main considerations for pregnant women planning longer flights?

On long-haul flights, especially those over three hours, there is an increased risk of deep venous thrombosis (DVT) in pregnancy. I suggest the following precautions:

1. Drink plenty of fluid while you're on the plane, and limit salty foods.

2. Carry out the usual leg exercises. Ideally, get up and walk around every hour or so.

3. Wear compression stockings and avoid restrictive clothing.

If you've had DVT or pulmonary embolus in the past, or have a medical condition that places you at risk, you should always discuss travel requirements with your obstetrician.

What about radiation risks to the baby from air travel?

The level of cosmic radiation in a routine long-haul flight is considered safe for foetuses. The oxygen levels in a pressurised cabin on a routine long-haul flight are adequate, and numerous studies have looked at the foetal response to these levels and have shown there are no concerns with routine air travel.

Pack the insect repellent!

Insect repellent—and its active ingredient, DEET—is safe for pregnant women. You should definitely pack some if you're heading to an area where mosquito-borne diseases like Ross River virus, malaria, the Zika virus and dengue fever are risks.

Pregnancy exercise: The third trimester

* Always listen to your body. Balance exercise with rest and relaxation.
* Add labour preparation exercises into your routine to strengthen your legs and keep your pelvic floor mobile. Try positions you may use in childbirth, such as squatting or kneeling on all fours, and work on strengthening these postures. You may want to do this at specialist physiotherapy prenatal classes.
* Keep up with moderate, low-intensity exercise that is within your comfort zone. If you're feeling up to it, continue to maintain your fitness up until delivery day.

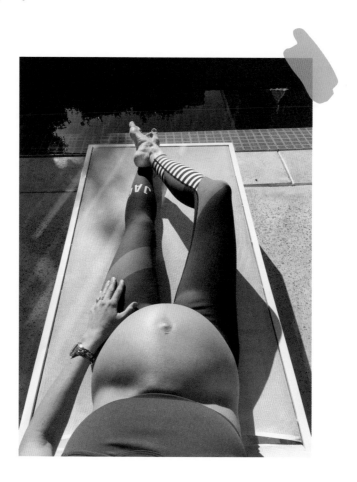

Interruption from an expert

28-week blood test

Dr Len explains the importance of the 28-week blood test.

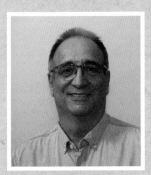

The Obstetrician
Dr Len Kliman

What blood tests are carried out at 28 weeks?

Around week 28 of pregnancy, you'll have another blood test to see if you have gestational diabetes. The blood test will also check again for the things we checked for at the first visit, to ensure that they are all normal heading into the third trimester of pregnancy.

Some women are at a greater risk of gestational diabetes—due to maternal age, family history, diabetes in a previous pregnancy, or some other risk factor. If that is the case, you'll be screened earlier than 28 weeks.

Packing the baby bag

. . . .

It's that time—time to pack your hospital bag. Seriously, the big event could happen any time from now. My doctor always told me to have a bag packed from at least 32 weeks, and even earlier with the twins. The good thing is, once it's packed you don't have to worry about it.

Here's a handy checklist for everything you need.

For baby

ONESIES
Yep, this little one is going to need clothes. Pack a heap of onesies (zip-up style, with the built-in mittens and socks). Bonds are ace for these, and they often have really good sales when you can stock up. *Do not* bother packing the fancy clothes you bought while pregnant and just cannot wait to get on your bub. The shock of caring for a newborn and adjusting to parenthood will have you tossing those clothes in the bin faster than your newborn can piss all over them (and that happens pretty much as soon as you take their nappy off). Those gorgeous twin-sets and mini sailor suits are adorable . . . but completely impractical, especially in the early days. Stick to onesies—they'll keep your baby comfortable and warm, and keep you sane.

BABY SINGLETS
As a rule of thumb, always dress your baby in one layer more than you have on—they lose heat quickly. This is especially true in hospitals, whose thermostats seem to constantly be set to 'dark side of the moon'.

BABY BEANIES
Again, these will help with warmth. We lose a lot of heat from our heads, so it pays to have a stash of these.

NAPPIES AND WIPES
While some hospitals provide these, many don't—check before you go. With Oscar, I didn't pack any nappies or wipes, assuming they'd be provided.

Newsflash: they weren't. It was a great start to my journey of being a Responsible Mother. Conversely, when I had the twins (at a different hospital), I packed about two months' worth of nappies and wipes . . . but the hospital provided it all. Bottom line? Just check.

MUSLIN WRAPS AND BUNNY RUGS

You'll be amazed at how many of these you'll need. Firstly, your baby will need to be wrapped most of the time (pretty much all the time, actually—except for when they're being changed or bathed). Secondly, babies are very messy (chucky, spitty, pissy, poopy) and you'll find that these wraps and bunny rugs are easily soiled. Pack around ten.

BIBS

As mentioned above, babies are *very* messy. You'll need a bib for each of the six feeds in a 24-hour period, multiplied by how many days you stay in hospital. Phew—are you beginning to imagine the loads of washing to come? Yep, babies are hectic.

For you

HIGH-WAISTED, BLACK NANNA KNICKERS

The bigger, the better! Heads up: you will not magically shrink down to your pre-baby size as soon as you give birth to said baby. I know, it is a complete rort. In fact, your belly will still be quite big, and sort of look like a half-deflated basketball for a few weeks to come. Also, your vulva will be pretty swollen if you've had a vaginal delivery. So you need (repeat after me) *big nanna undies*, like Cottontails. Even though I'd had two babies before, with the twins I didn't pack enough high-waisted knickers. Because I had a caesarean section, my normal-waisted undies dug right into my wound—the pain was excruciating. Go a size or two up from your regular undie size, and pack a lot. Like, at least four pairs a day. Because here's the thing: in the first few days post-delivery (whether you have a vaginal birth or a caesarean), you will bleed like you have never bled before. It will be like The Red Wedding down there. (And that's why I say black undies, FYI. This is not the time or place for your pretty, lacy, pink undies.) I remember pulling my pants down to go to the toilet after I had Oscar and seeing blood splatter out like in *Kill Bill*. It looked like a crime scene, but it was all completely normal. Still, it gets a little awkward when friends and family come to visit and need to use the bathroom. Lucky we're all so close.

BLACK PANTS

See above. Major leakage can (and probably will) happen, and there's also the (enormously high) chance of your baby pooing/weeing/vomiting on you. Choose pants with a high (but loose) waistband, so they don't dig in. If you have black maternity pants that fit the bill (like soft jogger pants or leggings), I recommend these (even though you'll want to burn them at this point). If not, go for loose tracksuit pants or leggings.

COMPRESSION WEAR (SHORTS OR TUBIGRIP)

Compression shorts are a godsend. Designed to support your abs, lower back and—ahem—nether regions—post-delivery, they also help get your tummy back to its regular, non-preggo state. I put my SRC Recovery shorts on as soon as I'd had a shower after delivering Billie and Oscar (and after medical clearance). Get fitted for your SRC shorts by a physio at 36 weeks so you have the correct size. If you don't have any compression shorts or Tubigrip you can ask to see the physio at your hospital after you've delivered, and they can prescribe you a compression garment. Post-twins, I had to wait until my catheter came out the following morning before I saw the physio who approved and fitted me with a Tubigrip. A Tubigrip was better in this case as it was easier for me to wear with my C-section wound. I felt so much better as soon as I put my compression garment on. They provide amazing support to your abdominal muscles and (if you have one) your wound.

MATERNITY BRAS

If you're anything like me, you'll need to start wearing these basically the day after you get pregnant—my boobs got so big, I swear they turned the corner before I did. If you haven't started wearing them, though, pack some for the hospital—you'll need them to make nursing more comfortable.

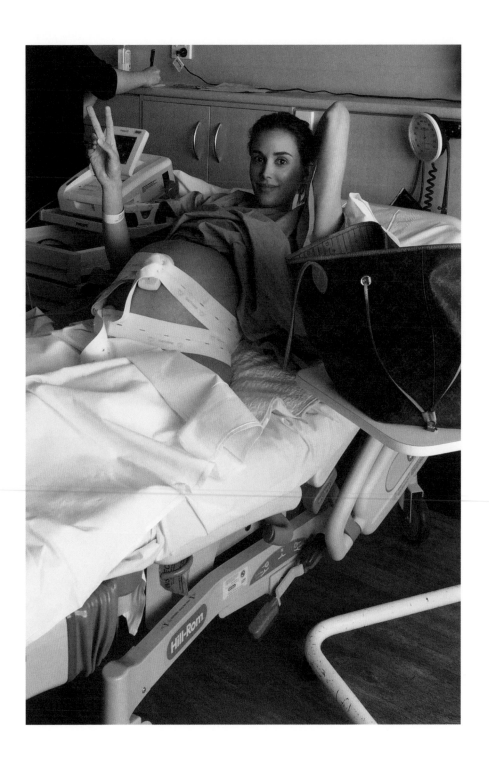

FEEDING TOPS
Choose anything that clips or buttons down—it doesn't necessarily have to be an official 'feeding' top: any top that's loose and easily exposes your breast (or can be lifted up) will do. Stretchy singlets are fantastic for this, and later, you can wear them under your 'normal' tops for easy breastfeeding.

FEEDING PYJAMAS
Ditto for PJs. I loved the button-down Peter Alexander ones—so comfy.

SOMETHING WARM
Pack a warm dressing gown or casual hoodie—hospitals get cold.

BREAST PADS
With milk comes leaks. Lots and lots of leaks. Pack breast pads to save yourself a slightly awks conversation with the orderly who brings you dinner.

TOILETRIES AND COSMETICS
While I didn't have the time or inclination to wear make-up in hospital, I still used an under-eye concealer (shovelled it on, actually) and pencilled in my eyebrows while I was there. I know, it seems a bit silly I suppose, but it just made me feel more like me. So while you probably won't have time for the whole shebang of contouring and so on (actually, scratch that: you *definitely* won't), if there's something you wear every day and don't want to do without, pack it. Pack your usual suspects, too: cleanser, moisturiser, soap (believe it or not, some hospitals do not provide soap), deodorant, toothbrush and toothpaste. I also highly recommend packing a good dry shampoo (I use Klorane) because washing and drying your hair in hospital is a definite no-can-do. Honestly, who can be effed?

MATERNITY PADS
Think about an amount you think is sufficient, then multiply it by three. That should do.

METAMUCIL OR FIBRE SUPPLEMENT

OK, so here's the thing: your first poo as a new mum is more terrifying than that time you watched *The Blair Witch Project* at a sleepover when you were fourteen. There are *stitches down there.* What if something . . . you know . . . *breaks*? It's scary but so much easier if you up your fibre intake. If you forget, at least eat all the fruit that's offered to you at morning and afternoon tea.

EASY SHOES LIKE SLIPPERS, THONGS OR UGG BOOTS

Don't worry, nobody judges how you look in hospital—make the most of wearing those Ugg boots in public.

YOUR BIRTH PLAN

If you have a birth plan, make sure to pack it.

SNACKS

While many hospitals have great food on offer, a lot don't. Pack healthy snacks like muesli bars, fruit, nuts and so on. Breastfeeding burns about 500 extra calories a day, so you'll be hungry. Load up on snacks.

WATER BOTTLE

You'll also be thirsty. Save the hospital a few thousand plastic cups and BYO water bottle.

KEEPCUP

You can have coffee again. *All* the coffee!

PHONE CHARGER

You'd be surprised at how many people forget these. And no, the hospital doesn't have spares. This ain't the Hilton.

SOME THINGS FOR YOUR PARTNER

Even if your partner isn't able to stay the night (say, if you have other children at home), they should still pack a change of clothes (birth can be messy for *everyone*) and other essentials, like their phone charger and basic toiletries.

Interruption from an expert

Third trimester ultrasound

This ultrasound is a really exciting one as it's now fairly easy to spot things like fingers and toes, and your baby is looking very 'babylike'. So what are we screening for at this stage? Dr Ngu runs us through what the third trimester ultrasound looks for.

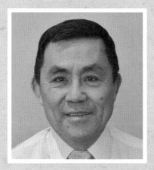

The Ultrasound Expert
Dr Andrew C.C. Ngu

What does this ultrasound check for?

In the last trimester, we scan the foetus to see if they're healthy, if they're the right size and to detect any additional abnormalities. When a foetus is too small or too big, there can be severe consequences. Foetuses that grow too slowly have a higher chance of suffering from long-term disabilities, including intellectual disability. In the case of a large foetus, it can be a sign that the mother may have diabetes in pregnancy or it can present a real problem for a vaginal delivery. Ultrasounds can estimate the weight of the foetus within 10–15 per cent. We also check where they are in relation to the placenta and cervix.

We also look for the amount of amniotic fluid around the foetus. This helps us to see the amount of blood flow to the foetus, which can reflect how well nourished the foetus is.

The ultrasound also gives the opportunity to check for abnormality. Very few abnormalities are found late in pregnancy (provided the second trimester ultrasound was normal), but sometimes abnormalities like hydrocephalus (too much fluid in the brain), dwarfism (short limbs) and hydronephrosis (dilated kidneys) show up.

Birth plan

. . . .

How do you want your baby to enter the world? A birth plan is a chance for you to write down your wishes about birth—the things you agree to do, the things you want to avoid. Sounds simple enough, right?

Somewhere along the way, birth plans got a little OOC and OTT. Making sure your baby comes out to the sounds of Coldplay? That's so over. I've heard of women writing down things like 'Make sure my baby is wrapped in a blanket that is gender neutral in colour' and 'Please use my scissors from home to cut the umbilical cord'. Look, we're all feminists here and nobody has to be wrapped in pink forever, but having a complicated birth plan can actually be a recipe for disaster. And those scissors from home? Trust me, you don't want them anywhere near your body or your baby.

So what does a good birth plan look like?

Basically, a birth plan is there to advocate for you when you can't do it for yourself. When you're between contractions and feel like you're clinging on for damn life, it might be tricky for you to say, 'Let's go on a little longer before we have an epidural.' So writing everything out first—and then circulating it to your medical staff—is often a good idea, especially if you have strong views.

I never really had a birth plan—I'm much more of a 'go-with-the-flow' person—but there are certain things I knew I wanted and didn't want. I wanted a healthy birth, first and foremost. If that meant I needed medical intervention—like pain relief, an induction or a C-section—then so be it. Having a healthy baby was my first priority. I was also adamant that I wanted pain relief, so I discussed this with my obstetrician beforehand.

If you would like to write a birth plan, have a think about how you'd like things to proceed—but don't get too bogged down in the details. Babies and bodies aren't always known for going by the book, and I reckon the more you fixate on a particular outcome, the more disappointed you're likely to be if it doesn't work out. That said, here are some things you might want to think about:

* Pain relief: yay or nay?
* Would you like to use the bath or birthing pool?
* Who gets to come in the room (both during the birth and afterwards)?
* Would you like everyone who visits the baby in hospital to be vaccinated? Add this to your plan and let the staff know, so they can play bad cop.
* In the event of a C-section, do you want to stipulate that the non-birthing parent gets to have skin-to-skin contact immediately?
* Would you like to speed up the delivery of your placenta? (You can do this via an injection.)
* If your pregnancy was complicated, or if you have special needs or religious wishes, be sure to include these so your medical staff is across them.

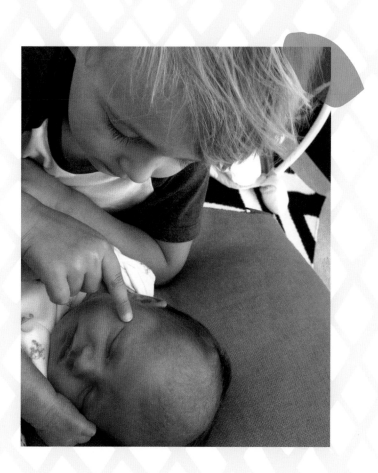

weeks 31–35

What's happening with baby

By now, your baby's sucking reflex is in full flight—if you have any further ultrasounds, you might just see your little one sucking their thumb.

Your baby is almost cooked, so the vernix and lanugo that's covered their skin up to now is beginning to disappear, ready for your bub to make their entrance to the outside world.

Another sign your baby is nearly ready? Their head will make its way down until it is fully engaged (i.e. in the right position for labour to begin). This may take some time, so don't worry if you see your doctor or midwife and they say your baby isn't engaged yet. It'll happen.

What's happening with you

You're big. Mate, you are so big. I feel for you. You're probably pretty uncomfortable by now—maybe getting breathless, possibly having leg cramps, almost definitely having trouble sleeping. (Which is just so cruel, isn't it? Like why can't nature just make us *hibernate* for the last two months of our pregnancies? That would be so much nicer.)

Size-wise . . .

Your baby is the size of a pineapple. So on-trend.

Month 8

Giving birth to the twins

Because of the potential complications with identical twin pregnancies, most women deliver early—from around 34 weeks. So for my pregnancy with Tom and Darcy, everything came earlier—the baby shower, the babymoon, setting up the nursery, finishing work. I stopped working at 28 weeks—and thank god, because I honestly could not move much after that. Getting off the couch was a big achievement. I was exhausted, sore and ready to have my babies.

Every week that went by, though, was a sign that my babies were doing well. Every week they were inside boosted their survival rate, and so while I was completely over being pregnant, I knew that it was best for the boys to be where they were. When we got to 30 weeks, we cheered. Then 31, and 32. By the time we got to 34 weeks, I was relieved and ecstatic—I knew they would be fine.

Did my waters break? Nope, I just pissed myself (again)

After 32 weeks, I started getting the most intense Braxton Hicks contractions. These are basically 'practice' contractions that help tone your uterus and get it ready for the real deal. Some women don't experience them at all (or else just don't feel them), but some women feel them quite frequently. With the twins, because everything was stretched to its limits and the boys' heads were resting on my bladder (thanks, guys!) every time I felt a contraction, the boys' heads would push against my bladder, and a little bit of wee would come out. It was mortifying. There were times when I'd wake up and there'd be a massive wet patch on the bed. I'd reach across to Chris and say, 'Oh my god! It's happening! My waters broke!' And he'd say, 'Nah, babe, you just pissed your pants again.'

The baby shower

If you've ever seen my Instagram, you'll know that I take any opportunity to have a party. Footy finals? Party. Start of summer? Party. New manicure? Party.

For me, having a baby shower wasn't about getting presents (in fact, I had a strict no-present policy . . . that nobody followed), but about having all my friends and family in one place before I popped.

These days, baby showers can be completely over-the-top—which is fine if that's your thing, but know that you don't have to do this. A simple afternoon tea with your girlfriends is fantastic. A lunch with all of your mates—men and women—is lovely. And look, if you don't want a baby shower at all? Totally fine.

When to have the shower

With Oscar and Billie, I had my showers around 34 weeks. With the twins, it was earlier, at 28 weeks. Basically, try to have the shower in the last trimester, but not so late that you won't enjoy it.

How to style the shower

While you don't have to go overboard with styling your baby shower, there's something nice about putting a little effort in to make your shower seem more like a proper event.

Personally, I reckon you can't go wrong with copious flowers, quirky balloons, neon signs, letter lights, cute servingware and beautiful stationery. Aim to have one central table for food and drinks, and style this area to add extra oomph and make it the 'hero' of the room. To add interest to your table, play with heights via tiered platters of goodies and go crazy with florals in vases of different heights.

For Billie's baby shower, we styled the room in a gender-neutral green and white theme. (Despite me having seen a vagina on one of her scans, we still weren't telling the world in case I was wrong—I mean, how embarrassing would that be?) We also used a 'B is for Baby' motif across the stationery, and echoed this with a huge B letter light on the hero table. We had these huge,

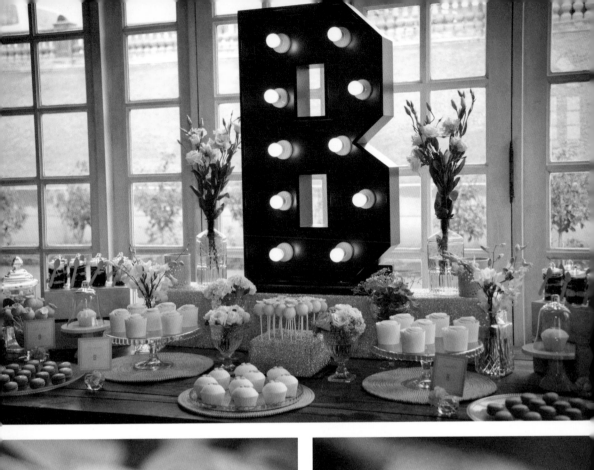

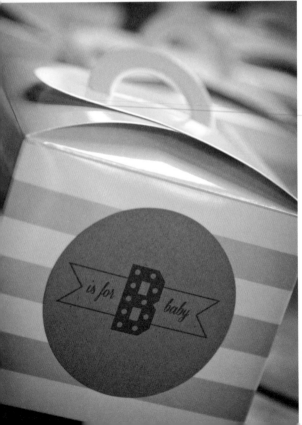

is for B baby

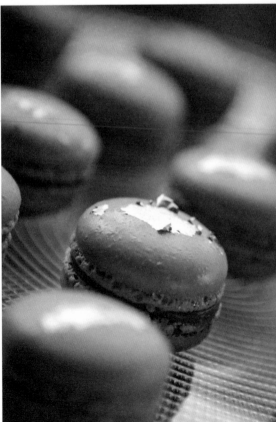

sparkly gold letters spelling out BABY in the entrance of the house, so it was the first thing guests saw when they arrived. It felt very fancypants indeed.

For the twins, we didn't want to do the traditional blue theme. (Not that there's anything wrong with that, but I did that with Oscar's baby shower way back when. Note there is no photographic evidence of poor Oscar's shower—it was BI: Before Instagram!) Instead, we went with black, white and green with a focus on fresh, green foliage and balloons. It was really striking and made a huge impact.

If you'd like to see the whole she-bang styling of the twins' and Billie's baby showers then jump onto rebeccajuddloves.com—you'll find the blog posts with all the pics there.

The food

High teas are lovely and make me positively fizz. Go crazy with tiers of cakes, biscuits, slices and finger sandwiches. Get your mum and your aunties and nanas on board and get them baking like mad.

I also love having one hero table laden with goodies. This way, people can help themselves to food when they like, and mingle the rest of the time. Pile your table with chicken and avocado sandwiches (always the most popular), pastries like sausage rolls and bacon and egg tarts, mini bagels and baguettes, cupcakes in all sizes and flavours, doughnuts (need I say more) and a feature cake. (I know, I know: it's not a bloody wedding. *But* the upside of having a big, beautiful cake is that you can freeze it and chop off slices whenever you like. We loved portioning and freezing our leftover cake and eating it over the next year for dessert. I highly recommend a chocolate mud cake with a rich chocolate ganache. It freezes well and when you thaw it, you can whack it in the microwave, heat it up and add ice cream. It turns into a warm chocolate fudge pudding, which you don't need me to tell you is bloody delicious.)

Serve the best champagne or sparkling you can afford. For the preggos, make a non-alcoholic punch. Mix sparkling water, fresh mint and lychees for the easiest version of this. If you're having a shower in winter, serve tea, preferably in adorable vintage teapots.

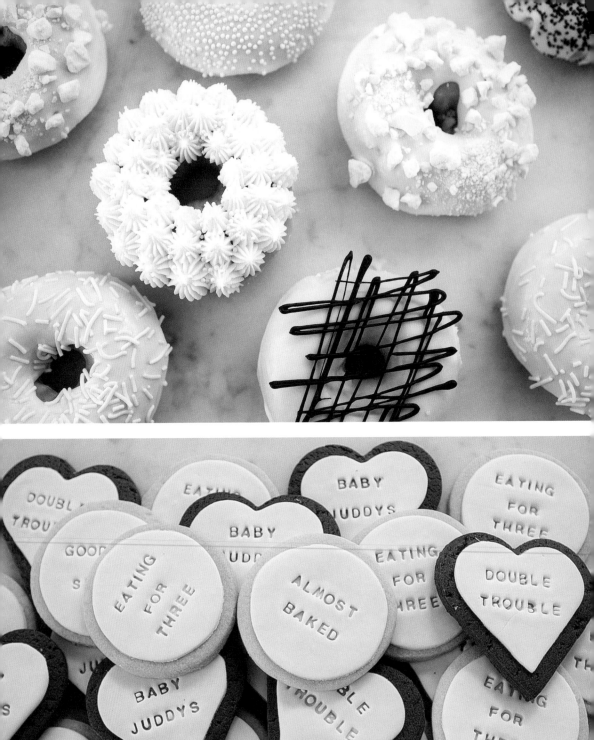

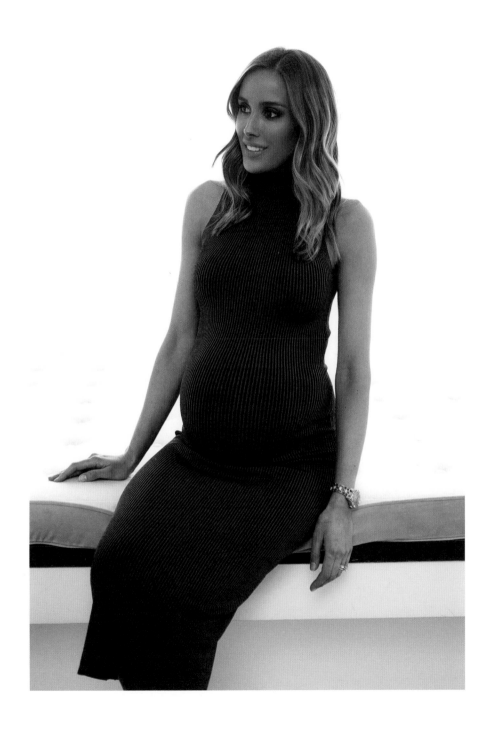

Baby shower games that you'll actually want to play

First up, let's get something straight: I would never, ever suggest you play naff baby shower games involving melted chocolate, nappies and a complete disregard for your guests' dignity. *Never*.

But even though baby shower games have a reputation for being almost universally cringey, a baby shower without *any* games can feel a bit . . . flat. So, here are my go-to baby shower games:

* Guess the baby's due date and weight. An oldie but a goodie.
* Baby Bingo—make a bingo-style sheet where guests have to locate someone who matches certain criteria. For example, 'find a grandma', 'find a mum with a newborn', 'find the mama-to-be's work wife', 'find someone who has twins', and so on.
* Solicited advice—buy a beautiful notebook and let each guest write down some advice for the parents-to-be.
* The Warm and Fuzzies—again, buy a beautiful notebook and let each guest write down a quality they hope the baby will inherit from the mama-to-be.
* Celebri-baby—print out some pics of celebrity babies and award a prize to the guest who can identify the most.
* Steal the Pin—each guest receives a safety pin to wear when they arrive, and the instruction that they are not allowed to say the word 'baby'. If you hear another guest say 'baby' you can steal their pin. The guest with the most pins at the end wins.
* Time capsule—ask your guests to bring a souvenir, photo, trinket or newspaper clipping of something huge that happened that year, or something that defines their relationship to the mama-to-be. This all gets popped into a box which is then gifted to the baby to keep as a reminder of what life was like when they were just a bun cooking in an oven.

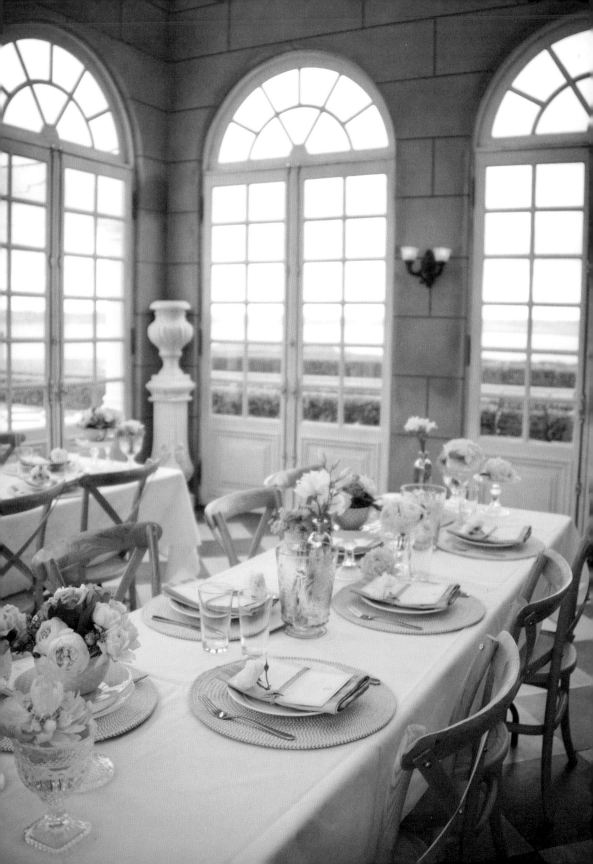

weeks 36–40

What's happening to baby

By week 37, you're considered 'full term'—from here on in, your baby could arrive at any moment. And that would be fine, because your baby is now ready to see the outside world. The brain and nervous system are fully developed, the bones have hardened (except for the skull, which needs to be soft to fit through the birth canal), and the lungs are mature, so that when the time comes, your little one can take their first breath. And scream. That's important, too.

What's happening to you

If you are quite sick of playing landlord to your tiny, unruly tenant, I don't blame you. Pregnancy is tough, man. By now you're probably carrying around a baby that weighs at least three kilograms, if not more—plus all that extra water and blood, the placenta, and perhaps a few kilos of your own weight, owing to a need for hot chips at hourly intervals.

I get it. Stick a fork in it: you're done.

Rest up, take a breather, get a massage, eat some more hot chips. You're so close.

Size-wise . . .

Congratulations! Your baby now resembles—in size only—a small watermelon.

Month 9

Nesting—and relaxing

By now you have been pregnant for almost a year (look, I'm rounding up because you deserve it). You are tired. You are sore. You feel like your pelvis might actually implode before the baby comes, and you're worried about how, in fact, the baby will be delivered if you don't have a pelvis. Mmm.

The good news is that, at this point, *you don't owe anybody anything*. This time, before your baby arrives, is just for you. Relish it. Enjoy every second. Not because—as people love to point out—when the baby comes it'll be harder to indulge yourself, but because you have just completed one of the toughest physical challenges on the planet. *Australian Ninja Warrior*? Give me a break. Nine months of having a mango-sized ball pushing into the top of your vag is far more excruciating.

So now is the time to relax. Unwind. Do things for yourself and bugger everyone else. Here's a quick checklist of things I did—and strongly recommend you get amongst, too.

* Get your hair done. If you need your colour redone, or need to get a treatment like keratin, now's the time. Just be sure to check with your hairdresser or doctor to see if the treatment is safe for you while pregnant.
* Get a manicure and pedicure. Make it the deluxe one, with the hot stones. And shellac, so it lasts a while. Who knows when you might get back?
* Take yourself out to breakfast or lunch. Every day, if you want. Why not? Order cake, too. Yes, even with breakfast. Again: why not? (And look, if you can't drag yourself out of the house, there are some recipes for goodies you can make at home on pages 128 to 135.)
* Go see a movie. In the middle of the day! Such a treat. You're going to spend the next ten years watching Pixar films, so make the most of this time.
* Get a facial. Not a treatment-heavy one, but a dreamy, hands-on, don't-mind-me-if-I-fall-asleep facial.
* And a massage. As above.
* Sleep in. I know sleeping is hard at this point (everything is hard at this point), but try to rest as much as you can.
* Read. Magazines, books, whatever—load up on them and read all afternoon long, if you so please.

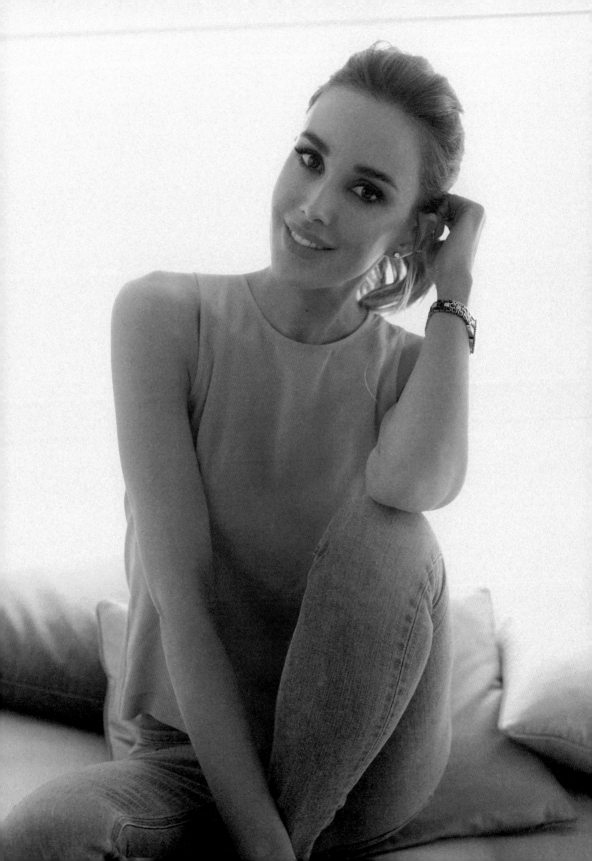

Setting up your home

You're 39 weeks in . . . and ready to pop. Before you do, here are a few things you should do around the house to prepare yourself for when you come home from the hospital with your new addition. And when I say 'things you should do around the house', I obviously mean 'things your partner should do around the house while you go get a massage and eat a large ice cream sundae'.

* Stock your freezer with carb-heavy meals. When people ask what they can bring you, or what you need, tell them 'lasagne'. And then tell them you are not joking.
* Make sure you have heaps of toiletries and non-perishable supplies so you don't have to do a big shop for a while after the baby is born. The last thing you want is to run out of toilet paper during a dreaded cluster feed day.
* Better yet, sign up to an online grocery delivery service.
* Set up mobile changing stations around the house so you can feed and change wherever and whenever. I would have a pack of wipes, a few bibs and some nappies in a few places around the house, so I didn't have to schlep back and forth to the babies' room every ten minutes.
* Stock up on antibacterial soap and hand sanitiser for every bathroom, and place a bottle at the entry of your home for visitors. There is *nothing* worse than newborn babies (and new mamas) getting sick.
* *If you haven't done this already,* be sure to tell friends and family who will be in close proximity to your baby to get their whooping cough booster well before visiting.
* If you have older kids, organise a roster of play dates around your due date. Even if you don't go into labour, you'll relish the time you can spend alone on the couch, watching a *Real Housewives* marathon and not *Pocoyo*.
* If you have noisy house helpers like gardeners or cleaners, try to keep them away for the first couple of weeks—both so your baby can sleep in peace, and so you can walk around the house with your breastfeeding boobs out.
* Have a sign ready if you have a noisy doorbell, telling people to knock instead. (Yes, you have become that person. Just accept it and move on.)

* Do a huge nesting spring clean before your baby comes so you don't have to worry about the hard house stuff until you're back on your feet. I'm talking: cleaning the windows, changing all the bedding, donating all of your unused clothes, bedding, homeware etc. Do it now and save yourself months of looking at dust on the tops of your ceiling fans as you breastfeed.
* Sign up for Netflix or Stan or Foxtel so you can binge watch TV when you're spending hours on the couch feeding.
* Download some audiobooks for middle-of-the-night feeds. They'll keep you awake but not *too* awake, and you won't have harsh blue light on your face or your baby's.

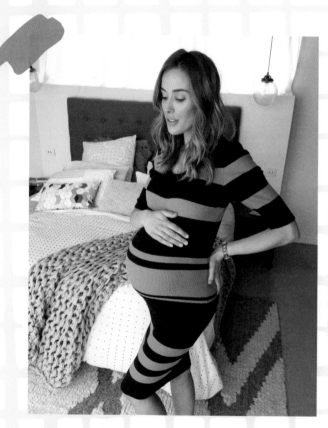

You know what they say about not wearing horizontal stripes? Ha! This is me at 31 weeks pregnant with the twins.

By now, you've been waiting for your baby for ten months. *Ten!* I know, I know: everyone says nine. But they lied! It's really ten. So if you were feeling proud of yourself before you read this . . . well, I bet you're feeling fucking fabulous now! You made it. Phew. Well done, mama. Now—let's go have a baby, shall we?

The
big day

Everything I know about labour

It's the Big Day. You've waited so long for your baby to arrive—and now bub is here it's bloody exciting and amazing and a teensy bit scary, yeah?

After three pregnancies, four kids and three very different labours, I've learned a lot about delivering babies. To help you prepare for this moment, here's what I can share with you.

Lesson number 1: Labour can feel like giant poo pains

Yep. Really. I was 39 weeks to the day with Oscar when I woke up in the middle of the night, feeling like I needed to do a massive poo. Which was so strange, because since when do you get up in the night to do that? The feeling went away . . . and then came back, ten minutes later. Mmm. I went to the toilet to check what was going on . . . and my waters broke. It was like a movie—suddenly there was this giant gush of fluids all over the floor. It had a pinkish tinge to it, which I knew (from all my obsessive googling) was what it should look like. It was official: I was in labour!

Lesson number 2: Sometimes labour makes you do crazy things

Like wash and blowdry your hair at 2.30 a.m., in between contractions. Yes, I really did this. No, I'm not entirely sure why.

Lesson number 3: Your waters can break—and then break again, and again, and again

After washing and blowdrying my hair, we were ready to head to the hospital. In all my first pregnancy naivety, I'd bought a pair of lovely, comfy Country Road tracksuit pants that I had decided would be my 'mum pants'. I put them on for the drive to the hospital, feeling very pulled together and prepared, not to mention crazy excited. I was going to have a baby! Like, really bloody soon.

As we drove on, though, it became clear that my waters were not done breaking. Every minute or so, I'd feel another gush of amniotic fluid. When we finally arrived at the hospital, my pants were soaked to the ankle, and the car seat was saturated. My poor, beautiful new pants were ruined. The lesson? Wear some old trackie daks . . . and a super-maxi pad.

Lesson number 4: Labour also feels like your bum is on fire

After five hours of contractions with Oscar, I opted for an epidural. I immediately felt a lot more relaxed (owing to the fact that I no longer felt like my insides were being crushed, I guess). I had a cup of tea and watched *Today* and did a bit of work on my laptop (yes, this is how good epidurals are: you can *work* while you have contractions).

Suddenly, though, something changed. It felt like my bum was on fire. Like it was burning. I called out to the midwife and told her, expecting her to rush me through to emergency, because surely it's not right for your *bum to feel like it's on fire.*

Instead, she calmly checked on the baby and told me everything was fine.

But everything was *not* fine. My bum was on fire! ON FIRE.

I called out again, and this time my obstetrician came down and checked on me. Lo and behold, I was 10 centimetres dilated. Oscar Judd was ready to arrive.

Lesson number 5: Sometimes babies have to come out really, really quickly

When Dr Len checked my dilation, he also realised that the umbilical cord was wrapped around Oscar's neck. This meant that Oscar needed to get out, *now*. Using a vacuum, Dr Len pulled Oscar out, as his heart rate was beginning to drop. It happened very quickly, and I hardly pushed at all.

I remember vividly the feeling of Oscar being pulled out—it felt like my insides were being pulled out of me along with him. On the third push, Dr Len looked at me and said, 'Get ready. You're about to become a parent.' I'll never forget that. A minute later, Oscar was in my arms: healthy, happy and totally ours.

Lesson number 6: Inductions can be great

When I was pregnant with Billie, her head had travelled so far down the birth canal that my obstetrician was like, 'She's going to whoosh right out of there when the time comes.' I had visions of being stuck in hideous Punt Road traffic, frantically trying to push this baby's head *back* into my vagina until we got to the hospital.

At my 38-week scan, Dr Len noticed that there was reduced amniotic fluid around Billie, which is a sign that the placenta is beginning to fail (the medical term is oligohydramnios). It wasn't an emergency as she was still completely fine (phew) but Dr Len decided it was best that I was induced a couple of days later, at 38 weeks and 4 days. I know a lot of women feel anxious about inductions, and I get it: the pain can be more intense. *But*, for me, it was a really great option. I woke up the morning of the induction, had a coffee, ate my breakfast, and calmly drove to the hospital, knowing exactly what was going to happen. No emergency roadside delivery for me! I didn't feel any of the concerns I had with Oscar—when will this happen, how will I know, will I make it in time? It all felt very normal, and made me feel like I was in control.

Lesson number 7: Epidurals are awesome

When I knew I was being induced with Billie, I booked an epidural. (Yes, you can do this. What a time to be alive, right?) I got to the hospital, had my epidural, and then Dr Len came in and broke my waters to get labour going. (As it happened, I was already 3 centimetres dilated, so it turned out I would probably have gone into labour that weekend anyway. But the comfort and composure that the induction gave me was so worth it.)

I've been told plenty of horror stories about epidurals (like the idea that the needle is basically the size of a sword), but for me, the experience was sublime. The only pain I felt was the initial anaesthetic that you have before the actual epidural, which was minimal anyway. And after that, I felt amazing. I was worried about having pain after delivery when the epidural wore off, but that didn't happen, either. I barely needed ice in my knickers. In fact, I didn't even need a Panadol.

Lesson number 8: You may not feel a connection to your baby straight away (and that's totally fine)

When Oscar came out, I felt nothing but complete shock. I knew I was supposed to have this feeling of overwhelming, intense love . . . but I didn't.

What's wrong with me, I wondered. Isn't this supposed to be kicking in? Aren't I meant to feel like a lion with her cub?

That feeling came later with Oscar, and I wish I'd known at the time that this is completely normal. Instead, I stressed that I didn't love my baby the way I thought I should.

With Billie and the twins, I did get that feeling of crushing, crazy love, and it truly is indescribable. I'm so glad I got to experience that, because nothing compares. It was like an old Disney cartoon—birds chirping, orchestra playing. I fell in love fast and hard. It was utter, utter bliss.

But if you don't feel that right away, don't despair. You will feel it eventually, I promise. And when you do, it will be just as wonderful as you imagined it to be.

Lesson number 9: Even if you've given birth twice before, you won't always recognise the signs of labour

The night before my 35th week with the twins, I went to bed feeling a bit funny in the tummy—like I'd just eaten something hard to digest (uh, like two babies). I was also having painful Braxton Hicks—but they'd been painful for weeks so this was nothing new. The next morning, I woke up with an intense need to go to the toilet (you'll soon know what I'm talking about), and some mild period pain. Mmm, I thought. Maybe this is early labour. But, like, really early labour. I figured with symptoms so mild, I'd be having the boys on my scheduled C-sec date, which was the following week (at 36 weeks).

Nope.

I was due for an appointment that day anyway, and when I went in, I told my obstetrician what was happening, and mentioned that my undies felt a bit wet. He checked my cervix and swabbed me to test for amniotic fluid. Then Dr Len turned to me and said, 'Your waters haven't broken but you are in labour. You're quite dilated. We have to get these babies out now.'

WHAT THE WHAT?

Chris—ever so conveniently—was the guest speaker at a big footy lunch that day (it was two days before the grand final), so I called him and told him to get over to the hospital right away. He did—but because he was at a lunch with about a thousand people, everyone soon knew I was in labour (including my manager, who called me and said, 'Are you in labour? The media just called.' I mean, for fuck's sake: can't a pregnant girl get a break?).

Lesson number 10: When you give birth to twins, there's a small football team involved

Unlike my previous births, where there'd only been my obstetrician, my midwife and Chris in the room, with the twins, the delivery was considered high-risk. This meant that, in addition to Chris, Midwife Cath and Dr Len, we were joined by a paediatrician, his assistant, two midwives, two nurses, an anaesthetist and a second obstetrician. Seriously, we could have filled a footy team with these people.

Lesson number 11: You may smell your skin burning if you have a C-section

Look, by reading this book, you and I made a pact to tell each other everything. (Didn't we? If not, it's way too late now.) When you have a caesarean section, as I did with the twins, you may smell your skin burning as the doctor cuts and then cauterises the wound. It feels surreal and pretty full on to smell your own flesh burning. A bit like a barbecue really.

Lesson number 12: Having a caesarean is not a cop-out

Um, no way. Having a C-section, in my experience, was actually harder in some ways than my vaginal deliveries. I think we assume that because you're not pushing, the labour is somehow easier. Nope. Not a bit. You're lying there, waiting for your baby (or babies, as the case may be), feeling yourself tugged and pulled like a rag doll. I was mentally unprepared for this—I'd thought it would be easy—and I remember thinking, 'Whoa. I do not like this *at all*.'

The recuperation after a C-section is also full on. With Billie and Oscar, I could get back on my feet (literally and figuratively). With the twins, my pain was a ten out of ten for days. I was on all the drugs—morphine, Endone, whatever they could give me, I took. I had a catheter in and couldn't move around properly. It felt awful.

When I finally stood up and had my catheter taken out by the loveliest midwife ever, I felt like my insides were going to spill out through my wound, *Walking Dead*-style. When I had Oscar and Billie, I felt like my internal organs were going to drop through my vagina, but this time, I was seriously worried my spleen was going to pop through my wound. I couldn't touch my wound, or even breathe properly—taking a deep breath made me feel like I was going to split open like a purse. Eventually I agreed to use a wheelchair to get around, and it made everything a lot easier.

Bottom line? Having a C-section is *not* the easy way out. Women who get caesareans deserve a great big pat on the back. It's major surgery and it deserves to be treated as such. Thank God for modern medicine and my wonderful medical team.

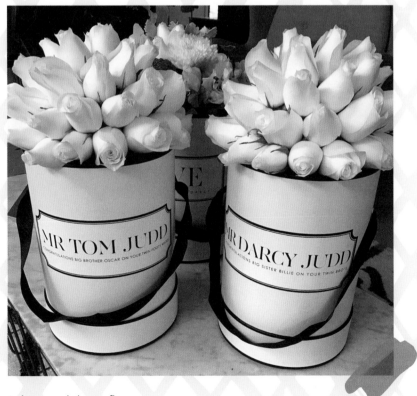

I deserved those flowers

Interruption from an expert

. . . .

Everything Midwife Cath knows about labour

OK—so now you know everything *I* know about labour. But I bet you still have a few questions. Luckily, my very own midwife, Cath Curtin, is here to answer them.

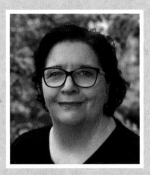

The Midwife
Cathryn Curtin

. . . .

How do I know I'm in labour?

Every woman comes into labour differently. To be in labour your cervix (the opening of the uterus) must be fully dilated (at 10 centimetres) to allow the baby to be born vaginally.

In the late stages of your pregnancy, you might experience Braxton Hicks contractions (BHC), which are painless 'practice' contractions. The difference between these contractions and true labour is that BHC do not dilate your cervix and they do not become more intense or frequent with time. Labour contractions, on the other hand, progress in both frequency and pain as your cervix becomes more dilated.

Signs of early labour include:

* progressive pain/contractions
* period-like cramps
* backache (this might be constant or come and go with each contraction)
* lower abdominal pressure
* indigestion
* frequent bowel actions (the day before or on the day labour begins)

* bloody, thick, mucous vaginal discharge (also known as 'the show')
* ruptured waters.

Signs of more established labour include:
* progressive pain with contractions
* vocalising with contractions
* strong lower body pain (with or without backache)
* ruptured waters
* inability to talk normally
* maybe nausea and vomiting.

When do I go to the hospital?

Go to your hospital whenever you feel worried about your health or the baby's health. You can go in any time during your pregnancy or early labour if something concerns you. As a courtesy to the labour ward staff, though, it's always best to phone ahead.

Head to the hospital during your pregnancy if you:
* experience bleeding
* feel unwell
* have severe headaches
* feel decreased movements from your baby.

In terms of heading to the hospital when you're in labour, there are many variables. Ring the labour ward and talk to one of the midwives—they'll be able to assess you over the phone to diagnose what stage of labour you're in. Make sure *you* talk to the midwife (not your partner)—there are questions only you can answer.

Going into hospital depends on the following variables:
* the gestation of the pregnancy
* the position of the baby (i.e. head first/breech)
* what number baby this is (i.e. if it's your first, you probably have time, but if it's your second or third, get moving!)

* if you are having a planned caesarean section
* if you have had any bleeding
* if your waters have broken
* how frequent your contractions are
* if you're having multiples
* your age
* your emotional state.

Am I supposed to stay at home as long as possible?

If you and your baby are well and you have plenty of support at home (and you've checked in with the hospital over the phone), it's perfectly fine to stay home until your contractions are about 3–5 minutes apart. In saying that, go to the hospital if you feel like you require extra support, or the safety and comfort of the staff in the labour ward.

Will my waters definitely break? What does it feel like?

Your waters (the amniotic fluid) can break any time during pregnancy, or during labour—or not at all. Sometimes the midwife or doctor is required to break the waters to help the labour progress. If you are being induced, breaking the waters is part of the procedure. As the vagina does not have a sphincter (a circular muscle that normally maintains constriction of a natural body passage) to control the flow of the water, when your waters break it feels like you are wetting your pants and have no control at all.

If you think your waters have broken, call your doctor or the labour ward to let them know. Have a shower and put on a fresh maternity pad so you can keep an eye on any further leakage.

The midwife will ask you what colour the fluid is, and how it came out (i.e. as a gush or a trickle). These answers help your medical team know whether your hind waters (slow leak) or fore waters (big gush) have broken.

If your waters have broken but you haven't started contractions yet, there are a few things that may happen, depending on your health and the health of your baby. You may go to the hospital to have your labour induced or your doctor may advise you to wait, watch and see if you come into labour spontaneously.

'Within the caul'

Some women actually give birth to babies without ever breaking their waters, so the baby is born within the amniotic sac—this is called 'within the caul'. It's extremely rare (occurring in just 1 in 80,000 babies) and is a pretty spectacular sight.

What if the hospital tells me to stay home but I want to come in because I'm feeling like things are moving quickly?

It's not a hotel booking, it's a hospital booking! If you would feel safer and more comfortable in the hospital, then that's where you need to be. You are the best judge of your body, so if you feel you are in labour, ring the hospital, explain your symptoms and ask to go in to the hospital.

What will happen when I get to the hospital?

Assuming you're not ready to give birth as soon as you set foot inside the labour ward, you'll fill out some paperwork (so be sure to bring your Medicare card, health insurance details and any other documentation you need).

A midwife will then formally admit you, fill in your paperwork and ask you what seems like a thousand questions (but yes, they are all relevant and necessary).

All your vital signs (blood pressure, temperature, heart rate and the baby's heart rate) are checked and recorded. If you have an obstetrician, they will most likely be notified at this point.

Then, it's a waiting game. As you progress, your midwife or obstetrician will check to see how dilated your cervix is and how far the baby's head is down the vagina.

Your pain relief options

Pethidine: This is injected into your muscle and absorbed into the bloodstream (meaning it also passes to your baby). This is a mild form of pain relief which helps you cope with labour, but does not take the pain of labour away. (Only two things do this: an epidural, and having the baby!) It can also make you feel nauseated.

Epidural: Administered by a specialist anaesthetist, epidurals are very popular as they're effective and have no effect on the baby. You may still feel pressure, but not pain. If you get an epidural, it will stay in place until the baby is born, the placenta is expelled and the staff are happy with your condition. After an epidural, you won't be able to stand (i.e. to shower) for a few hours, until it has worn off.

Nitrous oxide: Also known as 'laughing gas', this doesn't take the pain away, but it can help you cope better. It is most effective in the late stages of labour, when you're pushing or close to it. In early stages of labour, nitrous oxide can cause nausea.

What does a contraction feel like?

Your uterus is a muscle, and like any other muscle, it contracts and relaxes. Basically, this is what a contraction is. It's difficult to explain exactly what it feels like, but the rumours are true—it hurts.

Most contractions begin feeling like period pain. You may also feel a pain in your lower back.

Contractions come and go, and intensify as they go on. In early labour, contractions may come every 10–15 minutes, lasting just 20–30 seconds. As labour progresses and the cervix dilates, the pain intensifies and the contractions grow closer together.

When can I get pain relief?

You can get pain relief at any time. You can even get an epidural *before* you go into labour, if you want. This is a great choice for women who have a lot of fear or anxiety around labour and birth.

What, exactly, is an epidural?

An epidural anaesthetic is a popular form of pain relief used in labour that affects only a specific part of the body. The aim of the epidural is to give you a pain-free labour with enough sensation around the buttocks to allow you to push in the second stage of labour.

The anaesthetist injects medicine around the nerves to numb the pain signals to the lower abdomen and cervix, providing excellent pain relief during or even before labour. You feel pressure but no pain.

Epidurals have improved so much that some women can go through vaginal labour pain-free and have no stitches. Some women still go through labour pain-free, feel pressure but require assistance with the birth of the baby via vacuum extraction or forceps. Some women require an episiotomy or have a vaginal tear, but there are many factors that can contribute to this happening. An epidural decreases the length of labour and does not increase the incidence of a caesarean section. Don't believe anyone who tells you otherwise!

How is the epidural done?

The anaesthetist will fully brief you and your partner, while the midwife prepares all the bits and pieces the anaesthetist requires.

You'll be instructed to sit still, place your chin on your chest and relax by dropping your shoulders (easier said than done during the throes of labour). This way, the space between the vertebrae opens up to allow the passage of the epidural needle.

The anaesthetist washes your back with antiseptic solution and then injects local anaesthetic under the skin to reduce discomfort from the procedure. A fine plastic tube known as an 'epidural catheter' may be threaded through the needle, which is then removed. Inserting the epidural takes only about 60 seconds. Pain-relieving medicine is then administered through the epidural catheter and within 5–10 minutes the pain has gone. The epidural is then attached to a pump which slowly administers the medicine at a set rate. It can be turned down, up and off.

After the epidural is put in, a midwife will insert a catheter into your bladder. As you have no sensation you won't be able to pass urine. The catheter is removed after the birth when full sensation has returned.

The anaesthetist will stay while you have a few contractions to assess how effective the epidural has been. Often the anaesthetist will encourage you to turn on one side, then the other, to help the medicine work effectively on both sides. The anaesthetist will not leave until they are happy that you are out of pain and comfortable. If you require a caesarean section later in the labour the anaesthetist is able to 'top up' the epidural to ensure the lower half of the body feels no pain at all.

After the baby and placenta are safely delivered, the epidural catheter is removed by the midwife. It is vital you do not get out of bed unaided until the epidural has worn off as you won't have full sensation for a while, and you can hurt yourself.

When is it too late to get an epidural? When should I ask for it?

It's always best to get an epidural early if you want one. Labour hurts. It's the most intense pain you will ever feel and if you are going to have an epidural, there is no reason to wait until you are distressed and feeling out of control with pain. If you want to feel a labour contraction to tick it off your bucket list, feel one and then order the epidural, stat.

If you are dilated to 9–10 centimetres, it is too late to have an epidural. By the time the anaesthetist arrives and the procedure takes place you will be ready to push. So ask for one early.

What if it wears off?

If the epidural wears off, the midwife will contact the anaesthetist and they will come to see you and add more medicine to the epidural.

What if they can't get the needle in?

It is very rare that the anaesthetist won't be able to get the needle in. They do this for a living and are very skilled at their job. If they have trouble for any reason, they will try again. The risk of this happening is very rare.

Is the needle as scary as people make it out to be?

So much fear surrounds epidurals—mainly because non-medical people love to tell pregnant women information that is not accurate. The needles are not the length of a pole vault—it is a fine, small needle! The anaesthetist injects some local anaesthetic into your back (which feels like a bee sting), then all you feel is the pressure of the anaesthetist pressing your back to find the sweet spot to insert the needle. Trust me, you will be annoyed that you have wasted so many anxious hours googling 'epidurals' when the whole thing is over in a minute.

What are the side-effects of having an epidural?

* **Low blood pressure**: it's normal for your blood pressure to fall a little.
* **Loss of bladder control**: a catheter will be placed in your bladder as you won't have any sensation. Though rare, some women experience loss of bladder control after labour, too.
* **Itchy skin**: this is very common, as a reaction to the medicine in the epidural.
* **Feeling sick**: this is common, as your blood pressure drops a little bit and that makes you feel nauseated. The anaesthetist will give you some medicine to make you feel better, plus an IV to make sure you have extra fluid.
* **Inadequate pain relief**: rare and the anaesthetist will fix this problem.
* **Headache**: uncommon but it can happen. It settles.
* **Infection**: uncommon but it can happen. This is treated with antibiotics.
* **Temporary nerve damage**: uncommon but it can happen. It subsides.
* **Back pain**: common but settles quickly.

Will I still be able to push with an epidural?

These days, epidurals allow you to feel the pressure (i.e. when the head is descending) but not the pain. In other words, they are pretty much perfect in terms of pain relief. In most cases you should still feel the sensation of needing to push, and you should still be able to push when you are fully dilated.

How to push

* Try to relax: take quiet, deep breaths in between contractions.
* Focus on having your next contraction and pushing hard.
* Visualise your baby coming down your vagina.
* If you are sitting, hold your hands behind your thighs.
* Open your legs wide, letting your knees flop out.
* If you have an epidural the midwives will feel the contraction starting and tell you when to start pushing.
* When you feel a contraction coming, take a deep breath and push, holding your breath, right down into your bowel, like you are doing a huge poo.
* Curl up, pulling your legs open and push really, really hard.
* Keep pushing and pushing until you run out of breath, then snatch a deep breath and push hard again.
* Once the contraction has gone, stop pushing and rest. Take a sip of water, close your eyes and prepare for the next contraction. Remember, every contraction that passes means you are one contraction closer to meeting your new baby.
* When the baby begins to crown (i.e. the baby's head can be seen) the doctor or midwife will encourage you to 'puff puff puff puff' and not to push (to avoid tearing). Believe it or not, puffing can be harder than pushing!

I've heard I'm going to poo. Should I just prepare myself for that now? (And what do you do with it?)

Women rarely poo during birth, but before you push in earnest, you may pass a bowel motion (your body likes to make sure everything is empty). If this happens, your midwives or doctor will discreetly scoop it up and dispose of it.

We've seen it all before. Don't worry!

How is the baby monitored during labour?

During labour, both you and your baby will be monitored by a cardiotocography machine (CTG). The CTG monitors your baby's heart rate, the pressure of the uterus as it contracts, and the frequency, duration and strength of the uterine contractions. The CTG also assesses how the baby is coping before, during and after contractions. If the baby shows signs of stress, you may be induced into early delivery.

How long is a typical first labour?

Every woman labours differently. Some women don't ever come into labour and need to be induced. Like most living things, the placenta has a use-by date, meaning your baby needs to be born within ten days of the due date. Often induction is the safest way to ensure this happens.

Once labour begins it can take between two and twenty hours for the baby to be born. My advice? Don't look at the clock.

When do I start pushing? Will I know how to do it?

You start pushing when you are fully dilated, and not before (as this can cause your undilated cervix to become swollen).

And yes, you will know how to do it. The midwives and obstetrician will coach you through your pushing. Even if you attended birthing classes, in the heat of the moment you will still need some coaching.

If I swear at the midwife, will she forgive me?

Absolutely. I've been sworn at, put in a headlock (by the mother), vomited on, hit, had my hand squeezed until it turned blue, screamed at and much, much more. All is forgiven once the beautiful baby has arrived.

You might need an elective C-section if . . .

* You have pre-eclampsia (high blood pressure)
* You have a multiple pregnancy
* Your baby is in the breech position
* You've had a caesarean previously
* You have a maternal medical condition
* You are having an IVF baby
* You've had a previous traumatic vaginal birth
* You've had a previous stillborn or neonatal death of a baby
* You're of an advanced maternal age
* You have a very small baby
* You have placental insufficiency
* You have placenta praevia (i.e. when the placenta is at the bottom of the uterus, meaning it would be delivered first)
* You've experienced previous sexual abuse
* It is a medical emergency

What's the likelihood of stitches. Do they hurt?

The likelihood of having stiches depends on many factors, even your skin type. A lot depends on if it is your first baby, the length of the labour, and the condition of the baby and mother during labour. Having an episiotomy is basically a surgical wound, so yep, it hurts. It gets swollen and bruised, and like any other wound, it's going to feel worse before it feels better.

To help relieve the pain, take Panadol and Nurofen, and apply cool compresses. Have a laxative two to three days after birth so that you are comfortable doing your first poo after labour.

What happens in a caesarean?

An elective caesarean section is done prior to the due date (so the mother doesn't come into labour) and there is a medical, obstetric or social reason for the caesarean to take place. Once a spinal anaesthetic or epidural (or both) are given and the mother is comfortable and has no sensation below her waist, and both the obstetrician and anaesthetist are happy to commence, the procedure begins. The partner sits at the head of the operating table with their partner and within five minutes the baby is delivered via the abdomen. Yep—it's that quick.

The wound is about 15 centimetres wide. The baby is delivered by the obstetrician, often applying forceps around the baby's head to gently guide the head out. In a breech position, the head again is helped out by forceps. Once your baby is delivered, the obstetrician will quickly insert sutures and cover the wound.

What circumstances call for an emergency caesarean? What happens?

An emergency caesarean section is done when either the mother and/or baby are unwell and a vaginal birth may put either you or your baby at risk of illness or death.

Reasons for an emergency C-section

Maternal reasons

* Severe hypertension
* Other medical reason
* Undiagnosed breech
* Undiagnosed multiple birth (very rare)
* Failed induction or the cervix has not dilated
* Sudden collapse
* Sudden bleeding
* Eclampsia (i.e. fitting during labour)
* Motor car accident and the mother and baby are at risk
* Drug/alcohol overdose

Baby reasons

* Foetal distress
* Decreased heart rate
* Meconium passed (first bowel action)
* A limb presenting, like an arm or a leg
* The cord has prolapsed (come out vaginally)
* Decreased amniotic fluid
* Decreased foetal movement

An emergency C-section is the same as an elective one once it has commenced. You'll be given anaesthetic and then surgery will begin. Again, the procedure is very quick—you'll be seeing your baby within five minutes or so.

What happens right after the birth?

Once the baby is delivered the cord is clamped and cut, and the baby is handed to a paediatrician. The paediatrician then shows the baby to the new parents and along with the partner takes the baby to a warm cot. Your baby will receive a vitamin K shot (to enable blood clotting), an immunisation injection, a name tag (be sure to check it!) and will be weighed. Then, all going well, you'll get your baby back for the first feed and a cuddle.

Your midwife will check your health—blood loss, your pain level and, if you've had an epidural, how fast it's wearing off. Your baby's temperature will be taken frequently, to ensure they are warm enough. You'll be given pain relief so that when the spinal anaesthetic and/or epidural has worn off there is adequate pain relief (particularly with a caesarean section, which is major abdominal surgery). Once both you and your baby are stable, you'll be transferred to the postnatal ward.

When I've had my baby (YESSSSSSSS!!!!!), what will happen?

While you're in hospital it is time to recover, feed your baby (and yourself! You'll be hungry) and receive guidance from the midwives about the care of your baby. You will be offered pain relief and assistance with breastfeeding, changing nappies and bathing the baby. The midwives are there to help you, so ask questions. Remember that every midwife is different and some may offer conflicting advice. Go with your gut.

Depending on the birth, your health and the baby's health (and how many children you've had previously), you might be able to go home as little as 24 hours after birth. Many women opt to stay longer, especially in the case of a first birth. Don't feel pressured to go home, or to stay—again, go with your gut (as well as the advice of your doctor, of course). Enjoy those days in hospital— things will get a little harder when there are no midwives around!

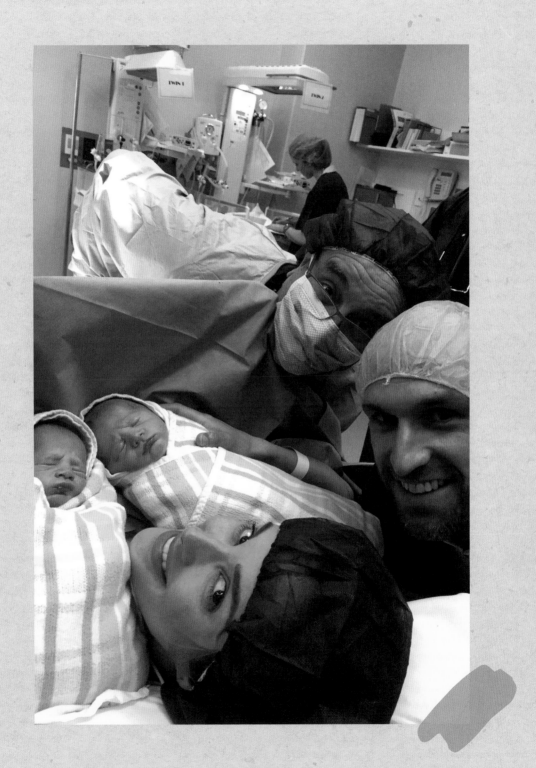

Hey, mama! You did it. You really did it. You had a goddamn baby. You. Are. Amazing.

But . . . as life-changing and challenging as pregnancy was—and as physically and emotionally exhausting as labour was—man, they've got nothing on actually, you know, being a parent. Your first few days—and nights—as a mum will be tough (as well as blissful, it has to be said), so I'm gonna hold your hand, and help you through. Let's do it.

Your first few days as a mum

Breastfeeding (or, how to use your boobs to keep your baby alive)

When I had Oscar, I just assumed I'd be able to breastfeed him. Like, milk would come out, he would drink it, and we'd be sorted. Happy days.

But it turned out Oscar was not too keen on my boobs. Initially, he was all for it. As soon as he was out, he jumped on my boob straight away—it was a bit shocking, really! I'd just delivered this baby and then—bam!—he starts feeding right away. The midwife told me I was a natural, but truth be told, I hadn't done anything—I'd just laid there, and Oscar knew exactly what to do.

By the second day, though, my boobs were killing me. They were completely engorged and so, so sore—they looked like giant veiny balloons filled with concrete. Every time Oscar latched on, I yelped with pain. Once he finished, *he* would start crying, which made me wonder if he was getting enough to eat (spoiler: he wasn't). And the whole time, all I could think was, *Hang on, isn't this supposed to be the most natural thing in the world? Aren't I meant to do this every day for like, a year?* At that point, the thought of doing it for one more day was agony. I didn't understand how some women made it look so easy. Nobody had ever—ever—let on that breastfeeding might actually be difficult.

I was at my wit's end. I was trying to do everything, and nothing was working. I wanted the best for my baby . . . but I felt like I couldn't even fulfil this basic need. I was exhausted, overwhelmed and bloody over it. Then I went to see Midwife Cath, and—halle-fucking-lujah—she said the words that I'd been waiting to hear (even if I didn't quite know it at the time): 'Your milk's not in properly. Your baby is crying. You need to top him up with formula.'

There is a lot of stigma around formula feeding babies, and I was not immune to it. At first I resisted Cath's ideas; I really wanted to stick with breastfeeding. But after giving Oscar a bottle and seeing him down it in 30 seconds flat (as opposed to the way he would suck at my boob for 40 minutes and *still* be crying with hunger afterwards), I knew that she was right. So I started to top Oscar's feeds up with formula (I would breastfeed, and then give him a bottle afterwards to make sure he wasn't hungry), and—whaddya know?—he became a helluva lot happier (probably 'cos he wasn't *starving*) and so did I.

'So, are you breastfeeding?'

When you have a baby, people will feel like they are entitled to all sorts of information about that baby, and how you plan to raise it. One of the most popular questions is, 'So, are you breastfeeding?' Let's get one thing straight: this is none of their business. People asked me this all the time, and I just could not believe it. It can be really confronting to have people ask you details like that—especially if you are quite a private or shy person. Like I said before, there's a lot of bias around feeding, too—so I felt like (with Oscar, anyway), if I told people I wasn't breastfeeding, they'd judge me. Ugh, it was exhausting! I wish I'd had the courage to tell people to sod off back then, but sadly, I didn't. But take it from me: you owe these people nothing. I'd recommend answering with either, 'That's none of your business', or simply changing the subject. 'Gee, the weather is *so nice* today, isn't it?'

Then, when Oscar was two weeks old, he was diagnosed with reflux. I remember sitting on the couch, alone (Chris was in Perth playing footy—lucky bastard), and trying to get this baby to feed. He would take a little, and then throw his head back and scream. At one point, I wondered who had cried more tears: him, or me? I felt like my boobs were producing poison—and of course, that made me feel like the worst mum in the world. It wasn't a super happy time.

At six weeks, I got a shocking case of mastitis—honestly, you wouldn't wish it on your worst enemy. At that point, I knew Oscar needed to be bottle-fed—it just wasn't working for either of us. After he started drinking formula—and after I'd recovered from mastitis—things really started to turn around for us.

While the benefits of breastfeeding are undisputed (for mum and baby), and while it's *always* worth giving it a go, sometimes—for many reasons—

breastfeeding just does not work. It was a huge relief to hear that I had tried everything—expressing, different positions, changing my diet (I'd even given up coffee!)—but it just wasn't going to work. It wasn't me, it wasn't Oscar: breastfeeding just wasn't for us. I felt guilty about ending breastfeeding—after all, every message you get from midwives, doctors and the public health system is that 'breast is best'. And it is. But sometimes it just doesn't work. As guilty as I felt, I also felt like a load had been lifted off my shoulders when I stopped feeding. As new mums, we have so much to worry about—in the end I decided to worry about whether my child was starving, not whether I was breastfeeding him or not.

Later, I breastfed Billie successfully (and effortlessly—wtf?). It was an amazing experience. Honestly, she fed so easily, I couldn't quite believe they were the same boobs! Again, I had Midwife Cath's unwavering support and guidance, which I'm so happy to share with you here. I quizzed Cath on breastfeeding—basically, this is everything you wanted to know but weren't quite sure how to ask. I hope it's as helpful to you as it was to me.

P.S. How bloody great are boobs?

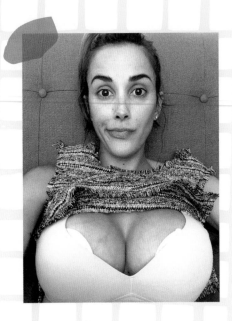

Those boobs!

Interruption from an expert

Everything you wanted to know about breastfeeding (but didn't want to ask in your prenatal classes)

Midwife Cath explains the ins and outs of breastfeeding.

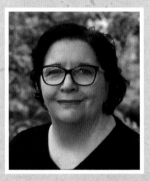

The Midwife

Cathryn Curtin

Will my baby breastfeed straight away?

Yes! Newborn babies are amazing. Many of them have been sucking away at their fingers, fists, hands or thumbs in utero, and continue to put their fingers to their mouths for quite a few months after birth. It is not uncommon to see a 'sucking blister' on a hand of a baby who has been sucking away while growing and enjoying life inside the uterus.

When your baby comes out, they will be wide-eyed, looking around to see what the world is going to offer. Hopefully, this is a boob. Newborns have a strong sucking reflex and your baby will be ready to suck immediately. When you are both ready, hold your baby close to your nipple, and let them search and find your nipple to suck. It may take some time, so be patient. Many factors affect the first breastfeed—for instance, the type of birth you had, how you feel, how your baby feels—so don't become worried if the first feed doesn't go 'according to plan'. It sounds easy, but like everything, breastfeeding takes time and a lot of practice.

Ideally, the first feed will be within the first minutes after the birth, but this isn't always possible. (A lot is going on, after all— the placenta needs to be expelled, you may need stitches, your sheets might need to be changed.) If you intend to breastfeed, it is important to offer the breast within the first hour. Babies are alert within the first few hours and they will suck and suck and suck. Then, after a nice feed, they hibernate and have a really good sleep. (And you should, too!) If you don't intend to breastfeed, give the baby a bottle of formula straight after birth.

How do I hold my baby to feed? Are there different positions?

There are different positions, but the most comfortable position (in my opinion and experience), is simply to hold your baby across your chest, with the baby's head in your left elbow (that's if you're feeding from the left breast; vice versa for the right). Hold your nipple gently with your fingers, making a peace sign. The index finger should be above your nipple and your middle finger under your breast, holding your breast up (especially if you have large breasts). Allow your baby to do the work and find the nipple. Honestly, babies are so clever. You do not need to teach a baby how to breastfeed. Trust me: your baby wants to live. Babies are hardwired to feed, not hardwired to starve.

If you have twins, use the football hold (sometimes known as the underarm hold), where you cradle a baby in each of your arms, as you would a football. This position is tricky to maintain, though, so I do suggest leaving it to mums of twins (and footballers), unless you really like the football hold.

How do I get my baby to latch?

The best way for your baby to attach is to let them find the nipple themselves. There is really no need for anyone to push the baby towards the nipple or hold the baby's head in a particular way. (In fact, babies *hate* this!) Babies want to suck. When you are holding your baby close to you, they will 'root around' and find your nipple. Trust your baby. Trust your body. And relax!

When will my milk come in?

Lactation takes about six weeks to establish. The initial filling of the breasts—what we refer to as 'the milk coming in'—takes place on a different day for every woman. Some women have fully leaking colostrum prior to birth, some get this on day one, some take a few days longer. In fact, some women never even feel their breasts fill—but they are still able to successfully breastfeed. On average, most women feel 'their milk coming in' between the second and seventh days.

Lots of mothers worry they won't make any milk. Remember that lactation of your breasts is a given. Your body knows it needs to lactate. Once your baby is born, the placenta is delivered and your brain knows to trigger the body to make milk to feed the baby. You don't need to take, eat or smell anything to stimulate your breasts as lactation is a brain function. All you need is to hold your baby close to you and let the baby suck on your nipple.

When the baby sucks on your nipple it stimulates a hormone to let down the milk into your breasts. It doesn't matter if you have small breasts or large breasts. Even women who live in much tougher places, with less access to food and water, can still make food for their newborn baby.

Everyone lactates differently, and it's important that women understand this. Not everyone has a huge amount of milk. Over my years helping women with lactation, I have seen women with so much colostrum that the baby is gulping colostrum straight after birth. I've also seen women who produce very little milk, and sadly it is just how you are made. This can cause anxiety and grief, as the mother wants to nourish her baby.

What is colostrum?

Colostrum is the first milk of the lactation. There's usually only a small volume of colostrum but it is rich in calories and also acts as an initial laxative for the baby. Even if you don't plan on breastfeeding long-term, nursing for at least the first few days is very beneficial, as your baby will reap the benefits of this highly nutritious milk.

My breasts are engorged like crazy. HELP.

When your milk comes in, you need three things:

1. a well-fitting nursing bra

2. pain medication (Panadol or Nurofen)

3. a baby you can feed as often as possible.

When your milk comes in—after about three or four days—you may have very sore, hard and engorged breasts. This can be painful but is very normal. It's called engorgement, and it happens when your milk comes in too quickly. The result? Hot, throbbing breasts that are painful to the touch, and very little milk to show for it.

To ease the pain of engorgement, I often use an old-fashioned natural remedy—cabbage leaves. Believe it or not, cabbage can help reduce the swelling and inflammation associated with engorgement. The only downside is you may never want to eat cabbage again.

Using a fresh cabbage, take off all the leaves and soak them in clean cool water to remove any dirt. Separate the leaves and place them in the freezer to cool (they don't need to be frozen). Place the leaves around your breast, avoiding the nipple. You can wear a bra or singlet over the top.

As soon as the cabbage leaves become hot and soft, remove them and replace them with new leaves from the freezer. (Hint: you might need to stock up on cabbages.) Take some Panadol or

Nurofen to help with the pain, too, and try to rest as much as you can (I know, it's not easy).

With engorgement can also come flat nipples, which can make it difficult for your baby to suck. Wearing a nipple shield can help to remedy this.

If you have sore, full breasts, try not to express—this will only cause milk production to be increased. It's better to allow your baby to feed as often as they like, as this will help create a sustainable pattern of feeding.

What is cluster feeding? Is it normal? When does it happen and how long does it last?

Cluster feeding is a term given to a 'constant session of breastfeeding'—that is, the baby seems to feed, feed and then feed some more, until it feels like you have been feeding them almost continuously for hours. This usually occurs in the early evening (what we call 'the witching hour'—between 5 and 10 p.m.), and it is completely normal.

There is a reason behind cluster feeding—it provides the baby with a volume of milk to prepare for the night sleep ahead. So even though it can be (literally) draining, it's always good to let your baby cluster feed. Remember, you cannot overfeed your baby with breast milk, so go for it.

How often will my baby feed in a 24-hour cycle and for how long?

All babies are different and therefore feed differently. Some may feed five to six times a day, some may feed ten to twelve times a day. Both are normal—for the individual baby. It's best not to time or have strict feeding times for a newborn baby; instead, try to respond to their needs. The frequency and duration of feeds will also depend on whether you're bottle-feeding or breastfeeding, the time of the day, and the weather (babies need more milk during hot weather).

Do I need to alternate boobs?

Yes, you do. It's important to alternate breasts during a feed to keep the milk moving. Feeding from one side only can lead to mastitis as the brain does not discriminate when it lets down the milk into the breast. So when the baby starts to suck and the brain lets the milk down (ejection of the milk), it lets it down to both breasts ... meaning your baby needs to feed from both sides. This will also help keep up your supply.

Why am I so hungry when I'm breastfeeding?

Good question! OK—let's say your baby was 3.5 kilograms at birth. By six months, your baby is capable of growing to 9 kilograms. The only thing helping your baby grow? The mother's calories, through breast milk. Your body is giving another person their only form of energy, which means you have far greater energy needs than normal, causing you to eat a lot more. It's remarkable. (What's even more remarkable is that, despite all your extra eating, you won't gain weight. Bring on the ice cream!)

My baby is refusing the breast—why?

There are so many answers to this question. It depends on the baby, their weight, their gestational age (i.e. the number of weeks they spent in the womb), the amount of milk you have and the size of your nipples. Here's what I know:

* Babies who wake frequently at night and have lots of breastfeeds tend to refuse feeds during the day as they have fed enough overnight. It depends on the age of the baby, but it's always best to resolve the night sleeping first, allowing your baby to feed more frequently during the day.

* Some babies refuse or fuss at the breast due to their age— they're old enough now to become distracted by their surroundings. If this happens, take your baby off the breast, put them on the floor to play and start again later. Don't fight

the baby to feed—this can lead to feeding aversion. (In other words, even bigger problems!)

* Your baby may be sick. If your baby is unwell, they may refuse the breast. Always check your baby's temperature, have a doctor check their throat and try paracetamol if you think your baby might be in pain.

* Premature babies who have some sucking issues at birth may experience some breast refusal.

* Some babies refuse one breast only—this is usually down to personal preference. (Yes, this sounds odd, but it's true.) Don't let it worry you: a baby can successfully breastfeed from one side only, as long as this is consistent.

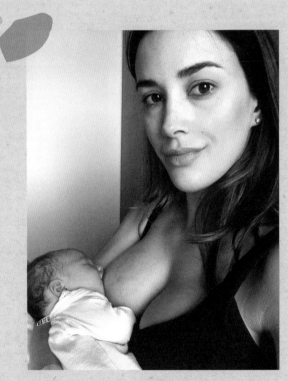

One-day-old Billie breastfeeding like a trouper. Check out my eye bags!

Do I need to express?

No. I only encourage women to express if:

* they have a premature baby
* they have a sick baby
* they have sore nipples and cannot put the baby to the breast
* they are going back to work early.

To breastfeed you do not need to express, although most women have expressing pumps on the top of their 'must buy' list. The best way to breastfeed is to let the baby do the work and not interfere with the milk flow by expressing. That said, some women who go back to work when their baby is under six months may need to express, if their breasts get full. If you do intend to give your baby a bottle, please see my advice below about introducing the bottle early.

What if my baby won't latch? Is there something wrong?

Some babies have difficulty latching for a variety of reasons. Often, the trouble is the shape of the mother's nipples. Trust me, I've seen thousands and thousands of them! Some are long, meaning the baby can attach easily and feed well. Some are shorter, making sucking a little trickier. Some are inverted, with the pointy part of the nipple going back into the breast. To breastfeed successfully your nipple needs to be sucked into the baby's mouth, so they are stimulated to suck, swallow and repeat.

If you don't have long nipples and can't attach the baby to your breast, I recommend nipple shields. These have actually been around for centuries, and are very, very useful.

While some midwives still believe nipple shields shouldn't be used, this is outdated thinking. Years ago, nipple shields used to be made of very thick rubber, which made it difficult for babies to feed. Now, they are made from a fine plastic that protects your nipple and allows your baby to feed well. If wearing a shield means the difference between breastfeeding and not breastfeeding, I say: use the shield.

Nipple shields can also help if you have sore or cracked nipples, which can be common in the early days of breastfeeding. You usually only need to wear them for a short amount of time, until the crack or sore has healed.

Though you may have heard that tongue-tie can prevent a baby from latching, this is not true. After all, a baby with tongue-tie can readily suck from a bottle (due to the length of the teat on the bottle encouraging the suck-swallow reflex). If you or your paediatrician think your baby may have tongue-tie, use a nipple shield to increase the length of the nipple, enabling the baby to suck and swallow.

What are the symptoms of mastitis? How do I treat it?

Mastitis is an infection of the breast that can occur when breastfeeding. It usually begins from a crack in the nipple, where bacteria can enter the milk ducts (it can also be caused by a blockage in the ducts). It doesn't affect every breastfeeding mother, but for some women—unfortunately—it happens frequently.

It is important to know the signs of mastitis so you can catch it early and start using antibiotics to treat the infection. First, you'll have flu-like symptoms—a nagging headache, sore throat, high temperature, hot and cold flushes, shivers and shakes, and a feeling of general malaise. This feeling can take over within minutes and you feel very sick, very quickly. Often (but not always), there is a red patch on the breast.

As soon as you have these symptoms, see your GP (if it's after hours, call a home GP—they bulk bill and carry antibiotics). You will need pain relief tablets, anti-inflammatory tablets and antibiotics—all prescribed by your doctor. Never take anyone else's medication.

It's very hard when you have mastitis, because you still need to feed your baby. Even though you feel unwell and your breasts are sore, you need to keep breastfeeding because the milk needs to continue to flow. It's very important to have the baby suck on the breast that has mastitis, even if it hurts. The feeding will actually help fight the infection.

You must not massage your breasts when you have mastitis. This is a common practice encouraged by some practitioners, but in my experience, massaging the breast actually makes things worse. After all, if you had a bruise on your leg that was sore and inflamed, you would not keep massaging it. It's the same with your breasts. If your breast is red, hot, swollen and sore, put a firm bra on, take your medication and let the baby feed. Clean, cold cabbage leaves (keep them in the freezer, as described on page 228) flowered around your breast will also provide tremendous relief.

The good news is, mastitis usually clears very quickly. Once you start antibiotic therapy, you should start to feel better within 24 hours. If you don't feel any change, go to your doctor or local hospital straight away as mastitis can form into an abscess quickly, and you can become extremely ill.

Remember to trust your body. If you don't feel well, tell somebody and get help.

What if I don't have enough milk and my baby is starving?

I see babies who are so hungry, they're crying constantly and losing weight by the day. The bottom line is, you must feed your baby. If that means using formula, then that's what you should do. Always offer breast milk first, and then top up with a formula feed (this can help extend breastfeeding). Breastfeeding is the best option for you and your baby, but don't let perfect be the enemy of good. In other words, if breastfeeding is not working, try formula. It is so, so important for you and your baby to be healthy and happy. We are lucky these days to have formula that is a genuine substitute for breast milk. Don't ever feel guilty about feeding your baby formula.

There's a saying, 'It takes a village to raise a child.' These days, our villages include preschools and Gymboree, but centuries ago, communities raised babies together. And part of these communities were wet nurses who breastfed babies if their mothers could not. My point is, every woman is different, so don't feel guilty if you can't (or don't want to) breastfeed your baby. At your child's 21st birthday party, no one will be discussing whether they were breastfed or not.

My baby won't take a bottle!

Even if you plan to exclusively breastfeed, you should offer a bottle in the first few weeks if you want your baby to be able to take it. Babies are very clever and know that if they refuse a bottle, later they will get a breast on the next feed. So introduce the bottle as early as possible, either with expressed breast milk, or formula.

I've seen many mothers try to introduce a bottle at three to four months—that is, when the mother herself is ready to head out alone again—and it rarely works. So my best advice is to give your baby one bottle a day within the first five to six weeks. This will not interfere with your milk supply.

Unfortunately not much can be done if your baby is older and refuses to take the bottle. You can keep trying (and hoping) but sometimes, it just will not happen.

Conflicting advice

The night after I'd delivered Billie, I was in the hospital, totally in the newborn-baby love bubble: adoring every second spent with her, sniffing her head and gazing with wonder at her little fingers and toes (seriously, how does something so tiny become so big, so soon? It's crazy). The whole feeding, sleeping, routine stuff was slowly coming back to me, but I'll admit: I was a little rusty on the details. After breastfeeding Billie, I noticed she was a little unsettled. I remembered I was meant to burp her afterwards (one of those things that just becomes second nature as a new mum), and confirmed this with a midwife who came in soon after. 'Yep,' she said, 'babies need burping after every feed.' Great, I thought. I've got this.

Later that night, Billie was still a little unsettled after I'd fed *and* burped her. There had been a shift change and I had a different midwife on. I told her how I'd breastfed and burped Billie but she was still crying. Perhaps she needed more burping, I wondered. 'No,' she said quite firmly. 'Breastfed babies don't need burping.' Ummmm, what? I was so confused.

One of the things you'll notice when you first have your baby is that *everyone has an opinion.* What's more, they will offer these opinions to you whether you want them or not. I guess people are just trying to help and have your best interests at heart, and there's something kinda nice about that.

But because everyone has their own opinion and advice to give, it usually conflicts with another piece of wisdom you've already been given.

Strangely enough, this conflicting advice begins in the hospital. Midwives, doctors and paediatricians all have their own ways of doing things, and their own knowledge to impart. Some midwives swear by dummy use, others throw them in the bin on sight. You'll hear conflicting advice about breastfeeding, sleeping and newborn routines. You'll hear from doctors who encourage as much skin-to-skin contact as possible, and others who don't see what the fuss is all about.

It's enough to make a new mama crazy.

My advice?

Go with your gut. Choose a midwife or doctor who aligns best with your values and temperament, and stick with their advice. You know what's best for your baby (even if you're overwhelmed and exhausted and entirely new to motherhood, you really do), so trust your instincts. If someone has given you advice that doesn't sound quite right, disregard it. And don't be afraid to stand up for what *you're* doing. After all, you're this baby's mum, so you're in charge. You got this. Trust me.

Visitors

Fact: when you have a baby, *everyone* will want to come visit you and see that baby.

This is lovely, of course: it means that everyone is excited for you, and wants to support you and meet the newest addition to your family. But it can also be completely overwhelming to have to deal with visitors when you're coming to terms with the fact that you've just pushed an entire child out of your vagina in the past 24 hours.

While everyone will want to come and see your baby, it's perfectly fine for you to set limits for guests. It's OK to tell people you don't want visitors in hospital. It's OK to tell people that you need to sleep, and that it is time for them to go. It's OK to say that you're not ready for visitors at all and that you'll let them know when you are (and it's OK if this is not for another six weeks. Seriously. It is OK).

Having a baby is a big deal. While your family and friends are no doubt incredibly excited for you, you get to dictate when they can visit, and how long they stay for.

You also get to tell them exactly how strong you would like your coffee, and what kind of cake you'd like them to bring.

Just FYI.

Baby blues

The first few days after giving birth are a blur of emotion. You'll feel insanely excited (after Billie and then the twins were born, I basically begged my husband to have another one immediately) and crushingly low. This is perfectly normal—you've just experienced a major life event, and your hormones are like dodgem cars, rattling around inside you, looking for a place to park. If you find yourself weepy one minute and laughing maniacally the next, don't worry—you're just adjusting to life as a mum.

When Oscar was born, I was on a high for about three days. I felt like I was running on adrenaline and, looking back, I was probably in a little bit of shock. First babies are so overwhelming. It's difficult to explain how overwhelming, but basically, I looked like the surprised emoji. All day long.

So there I was, navigating new parenthood (or attempting to, anyway) like a total amateur (which is completely normal) . . . when my risotto came.

Yep. My risotto.

Plot twist, right?

Still in the hospital, I'd ordered risotto for my dinner, and was really looking forward to tucking in (as any breastfeeding mum will know, carbs taste even better when you have a baby literally feeding off you). But when the risotto came, it was disgusting. Clumpy. Mushy. Salty. Gross.

So I cried.

Actually, that's an understatement. I bawled. I sobbed.

My risotto wasn't right.

This was a complete disaster.

Chris stared at me. 'What's wrong, babe?'

I couldn't even get the words out to tell him why I was so upset. I watched as my tears splashed into the sticky bowl of rice and just shook my head.

Later, I recognised that this was a classic case of post-baby hormones running amok. But at the time, I truly felt like my world was ending. (Yeah, over a bowl of risotto. I know how stupid it sounds, trust me.) When I had the twins, a similar thing happened—Oscar beat me at a game of snakes and ladders, and I lost it, sobbing over the board game this time, not a bowl of rice. Poor Oscar was so upset and kept asking me if I was OK—he must have thought I'd gone nuts. Luckily, by that stage, I knew enough about those first few days after birth to recognise that I was simply experiencing a hormonal wave and crash, and I was able to move on quickly.

When it's more than baby blues

I consider myself very lucky to have never experienced true postnatal depression. While I may have had a few days of postpartum baby blues, I never felt like harming myself or my babies, and I was able to get back into the groove of my life relatively easily.

For many women, though, this is not the case. Postnatal depression is real, and it is nothing to be ashamed of. Having a baby is traumatic, in many ways—it's a complete disruption of your former life, and it will change you in ways you've never dreamed of. It makes sense that something as challenging and transformative as childbirth can lead to feelings of inadequacy, sadness and even self-harm.

Not all postnatal depression looks the same

While I have never experienced true postnatal depression, my good friend Kylie Brown, who I met through football (her husband Jonathan played for the Brisbane Lions), has. She has generously offered to share her story of postnatal depression and anxiety.

When my daughter Olivia was born, the doctor laid her on my chest. I felt completely numb. I couldn't talk. I can't remember the beaming smile on my husband's face or even the moment I realised my baby was a girl. I felt like I wasn't really there, on the hospital bed. Something very strange was happening; I felt totally disconnected from the events around me. All I remember is lying there holding her and waiting for that feeling that everyone talks about: the overwhelming feeling of love when you first lay eyes on your baby and hold them. I waited, and waited, and waited. It didn't come.

Publicly, I presented a calm, happy facade. I had wanted to have a baby. And I had a perfectly healthy, happy little girl. I had nothing to be sad about. We lived a very fortunate life. Who was I to complain? So I went about my business, showing up to events with my friends, going to the park with my baby and so on. If you didn't know me well, you'd never have imagined I had postnatal depression and anxiety.

For the next thirteen months, though, I struggled with persistent physical symptoms that I later learned were manifestations of postnatal depression and anxiety. I experienced vertigo and dizziness. I constantly felt as if I was living outside my body. I felt weak and exhausted, even when I had twelve hours of sleep at night and daytime naps, too. My left ear was blocked. I struggled to do everyday tasks, like buying groceries, or even making my baby's breakfast—stuff like this would send me into a stressed-out spin.

I felt out of control.

Though I never felt like harming myself or my baby, I knew that something was wrong. It wasn't right for me to feel so physically defeated all the time. Eventually I went to my doctor. I had three CT scans, three MRIs, and two hearing and balance tests. I saw three different ear, nose and throat specialists, a balance specialist, two acupuncturists, two naturopaths, a Chinese doctor and three GPs to try to find out what was wrong with me. Everything came back clear.

But eighteen months after Olivia was born, I couldn't take it anymore. I'd seen the inside of so many doctors' offices, and had left them all without answers or even hope. I'd done numerous detoxes. I'd tried all manner of potions. I'd had more meltdowns than I care to recall. I was utterly exhausted, and scared that I was going to feel like this forever. I remember very clearly thinking, Make me feel numb. Put me to sleep for a very long time.

I went to my regular GP and cried uncontrollably. I tried to explain what was happening, but I'm not sure I did. At any rate, my GP prescribed an anxiety and antidepressant pill, and told me to come back once a week for an hour-long chat until I felt like I was back on course. From that day I began to feel better, perhaps because I had finally given in to my feelings, or perhaps because I knew help was on the way.

I get teary thinking about this, but that visit literally saved my life. Looking back, I know now how important it is to have a GP (or other medical professional) who you trust and can speak openly with. If I didn't have my doctor, who I knew well (and who knew me), who knows what might have happened?

If you had told me that I was suffering from postnatal depression at the time, I probably wouldn't have believed you. I think I thought that your situation had to be really terrible to have issues like that—but I had a baby who slept all night, took three naps a day and was healthy and happy. My internal self wasn't aligned with what was going on at home, but I had no idea it was postnatal depression. I'm so glad I got the diagnosis, though: it made sense, and it made me feel less alone.

It's been more than five years, and while I don't think of myself as 'cured' (after all, postnatal depression is not an infection—you don't just pop a pill and get over it), I do feel empowered. When I'm struggling, I know the signs. I know what I need to do. And for me, that is so, so important.

I want other women (and men, too) to know that postnatal depression and anxiety can present in so many different ways; some women tick every box in a list of symptoms, but some may not tick one. The most important thing is to listen to your body and know that if you don't feel quite right, there are so many people who can help you. I think some people struggle to see postnatal depression as a 'real' issue, as it can be difficult to see what is so hard about having a baby, especially when a mother has been desperate for one. But postnatal depression is real. Yes, there will always be someone out there who is worse off than you are, but that doesn't make your feelings any less real—and nor does acknowledging that make your feelings go away.

I also want women to know that postnatal depression and anxiety does not discriminate. I had everything I'd ever dreamed of—to everyone around me, my life seemed perfect. But I was not myself. And I was not coping.

Every motherhood experience is different, but we all deserve to feel happy and healthy. Please don't do what I did and wait eighteen months to seek help. Put your hand up and tell someone close to you: 'I'm not coping, I need help' or simply, 'I'm not OK'. The faster you do it, the closer you'll be to getting better and enjoying those precious moments with your children.

Symptoms of postnatal depression

* Persistently feeling sad
* Lack of confidence and low self-esteem
* Anxiety relating to your baby's health—for example, thinking they are unwell when they are perfectly healthy
* Obsessing over your baby's breathing, weight gain, routine, sleep etc.
* Persistent negative thoughts
* Feeling guilty and inadequate
* Irritability and tearfulness
* Poor or changed sleeping habits
* Anxiety, panic attacks and heart palpitations
* Loss of appetite
* Fear you might harm your baby
* Not bonding with your baby
* Feeling resentful towards your baby, partner and other children
* Taking no pleasure from being with your baby
* Taking no pleasure from things you used to enjoy
* Exhaustion
* Not wanting to see friends or family
* Suicidal feelings or the urge to self-harm

If you feel like these symptoms apply to you, see your GP immediately or go to **beyondblue.com.au**. Help is out there, trust me.

By the end of your pregnancy, you're feeling big and bloated and totally different from your old self—and if you're anything like me, you're probably imagining that once you pop that baby out, your body will bounce right back to its old self.

Mmm.

Not quite.

The truth is, it takes everyone time to get back to their old selves after they have a baby. Being pregnant is tough. It's a huge transformation: after all, over the last nine months, your body has literally made another person. Expecting it to fit into skinny jeans a week postpartum is a little much, when you think about it that way.

My advice? Go easy on yourself. Take time to rest when you can, and slowly (slowly!) work your way up to some gentle exercise—not to get back into those skinnies, but to release endorphins, catch some sunshine and experience what it's like to walk around without a giant bowling ball strapped to your belly.

Recovery

Your body after birth

About a year after I had Oscar, I went to get my moles checked.

You can just tell this is going to be a really scintillating story, right?

Anyway, I went to have my skin checked, which I do every year or so. The doctor took a bunch of photos of naked old me, and then compared them to photos he'd taken at my last appointment, which was before I was pregnant with Oscar.

Whoa. Big mistake. Huge.

I'd been feeling pretty good about my body—I'd started exercising again and could fit into most of my old clothes. Weight-wise, I was back to my old self. But looking at these photos of me, side by side, pre- and post-baby . . . there was no denying that my body had changed. Like, a lot. My boobs pointed a little more south than I would have liked, my tummy definitely wasn't flat and my innie belly button was now firmly out. For someone who—for better or worse—cares about how she looks, this was a shock to me.

The pressure to bounce back to your pre-baby body is huge. You don't need me to tell you that. It's hard to turn off negative thoughts once they're in your head, and it doesn't matter who you are or what you look like. Body image is not about how you look on the outside—it's about what you feel on the inside.

Social media can be cool . . .

But if you're feeling like shit about the way you look, get off it! If Instagram (or whatever) is making you feel down about your appearance, delete it from your phone. It's easy to get wrapped up in other people's social media feeds (which, FYI, are totally glossed up and approximately 65 per cent faker than their real lives) when you're not feeling so crash hot, so my advice is to ignore it altogether.

I'm going to be completely honest here and say: I don't know how to fix bad body image. I just don't. Your body has just done something entirely incredible—it has grown a baby from *nothing*, from a tiny speck of an egg you couldn't even see with your naked eye, and then it pushed that baby out and now, your body is literally feeding that baby and keeping it alive. If this were a science fiction book, you wouldn't believe it.

So it makes sense that, after doing all of this, your body will look different.

You might love your post-birth body. If you do, I applaud you. You should love it. It's yours—and look what you did with it. You're a bloody legend.

If, like me, you look at your post-baby body and wish—even just a little—that you could have your pre-baby boobs back, that is OK, too. But don't get hung up on the way you look. You're doing an amazing job. For now, that's what matters. That, and coffee. Always coffee.

What worked for me

After the twins (when I had a caesarean), my abdominal separation was 8 centimetres. I didn't feel great about that, let me tell you. I made sure I put my compression wear on as soon as I got the all clear from medical staff and embarked on pelvic floor and transverse abdominis exercises to help close the gap and get back on the road to recovery.

With all of my babies, I recommenced light exercise (and I mean really light) when I'd received the OK from my obstetrician and women's health physio. I can't recommend this highly enough. The good endorphins that flow through your body—plus the fact you're reclaiming your body—go a long way in making you feel positive about yourself. Personally, this certainly helped me with the transition to new parenthood—every single time.

Interruption from an expert

Caring for your body post-birth

The first few days after you give birth are full on. You're bleeding. Your boobs are swollen with milk. You're exhausted. Under any other circumstances, you'd be taken straight to hospital for complete bed rest. Except that's not happening, because you have a tiny baby to take care of. Sheesh.

Still, even though this time is very busy, there are some things you can do to take care of yourself. Here's Shira Kramer on the best ways to recover from childbirth (aside from, you know, having a stork deliver your baby in the first place).

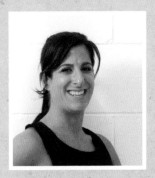

The Women's Health Physiotherapist
Shira Kramer

1. Rest and recover

In the early days after delivery, rest and recovery should be your main priority. Limit visitors as much as possible, and focus on yourself and your baby. You've just done something life-changing and physically exhausting—you need time to relax. Your pelvic floor and perineum may be bruised or swollen, and your breasts will be changing as your milk comes in and your baby learns to feed. Don't move around too much—it's imperative that you allow soft tissue to heal and your energy levels to recover before returning to any sort of exercise, even gentle walking. So for at least two days (and longer if you've had a difficult delivery or caesarean section), lie back, rest and allow your body to heal and recover.

2. The RICER principle

After a vaginal delivery you will have suffered soft tissue inflammation in the perineal area, so apply the RICER principle, just as you would with any soft tissue injury after sport.

Rest: Get horizontal and rest as much as possible.

Ice: Apply small icepacks or water-filled condoms (wrapped in soft material) against your perineum. This will help decrease pain and swelling. Apply for twenty minutes every two hours for the first three days post-birth.

Compression: Wearing comfortable (but firm) underpants with maternity pads can provide effective compression of the perineal area, which will help healing.

Elevation: Lie horizontally as often as possible, ideally face down with your pelvis slightly tilted (prop a pillow under your pelvis) to help reduce swelling and pain.

Referral: If you have any concerns post-delivery, don't be quiet. Tell someone immediately. It doesn't matter how minor it seems—say something.

. . . .

Getting back into exercise

When I felt ready to work out again post-birth, I visited my women's health physio, Shira Kramer, who gave me a once-over to make sure I was well enough to run, lift, jump and so on. Your body has been through so much, it's vital you get medical clearance before you start using it to exercise again. Here is Shira's guide to starting an exercise regime post-delivery.

When you feel ready, it's time to start exercising again. Staying fit and healthy in early motherhood has so many benefits—not just physical (though your posture, core, pelvic floor and back health will all improve with appropriate exercise), but also for your psychological wellbeing. Getting out for a walk every day with your baby can do wonders for you, your mood and energy levels. (And as a bonus: your baby will start to learn the difference between night and day the more you get out of the house.)

Don't start exercise until you feel ready and have the go-ahead from your doctor. When you begin exercising will depend on whether you had a vaginal birth or a caesarean section, whether you had pain relief, and whether there were any complications during or after birth. Some women are capable of resuming physical activities within days of delivery, while others can take weeks or even months. Be patient. Your body needs time to recover.

Most women can begin pelvic floor and deep abdominal exercises within a few days after birth, and can return to slow, gentle walking in the first few weeks. Don't walk for too long— half an hour is plenty.

After six weeks: Getting back on the horse*

There's a lot of confusion around when to start exercising after the birth of your baby, as well as what type of exercise is OK, and at what intensity. For up to a year after the birth of your baby, you're considered to be 'postnatal', and because of this, you need to give special consideration as to when to commence exercise. Even if you were a marathon runner before you got pregnant, you shouldn't simply lace up your sneakers and hit the pavement as soon as you give birth. Your body has changed and in many ways will still be recovering for months to come.

Why is it important to think about exercising again so soon?

It is vital to make a gradual return to exercise, to take your time and to listen to your body. We know that there are enormous physical and psychological benefits from exercising in early motherhood. You will not only look and feel better, but also have

* Not a literal horse. Not right now. It's not even time to go to spin class, if you get my drift.

more energy. There is also research to suggest that women who exercise in the first four months following delivery are better able to prevent or manage postnatal depression.

What should I do before I head back to the gym?

Before you head back to the gym, see your medical caregiver or women's health physio. Your women's health physio will check your pelvic floor and abdominal muscles before giving you the all clear to start exercising again.

What sort of exercise is best for me?

After the first six weeks, low-impact options are the way to go. Gradually increase your walking by building up distance and speed. (Bonus: most babies love sleeping in the pram. Embrace it.) Swimming, cycling, postnatal (or Clinical) Pilates or other postnatal classes are other great ways to start. You could also find a program that allows you to integrate your baby into your exercise, like a postnatal program or mums and babies yoga class. Strength and conditioning can generally start at six weeks, but wait at least three to six months before commencing more intense, higher impact exercise such as aerobics, tennis and running.

Protect your back

Lift nothing heavier than your baby for at least six months after delivery to ensure that your pelvic floor and deep abdominals can recover properly.

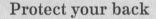

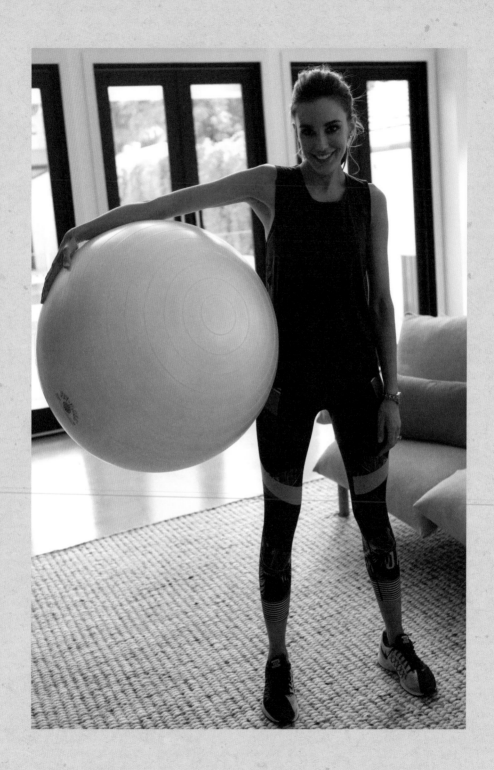

How long will it take to get fit again?

I see a lot of women who are really keen to get back to their pre-baby bodies. They want instant results and become unhappy when their body doesn't do what they expect it to. It is so important for new mums to be patient and listen to their bodies when it comes to postnatal exercise. Don't expect your body to return to normal soon after your baby arrives—your body has changed, and it takes time and work to lose weight and recover. If you rush to get back into your jeans, you may inadvertently put your body at risk of injury, and hinder rather than help your recovery. Remember to be kind to yourself—give yourself a chance to heal. Realistic goals based on understanding and listening to your body will optimise the quality and speed of your recovery.

Fact: nothing is as terrifying as strapping your baby into the car seat for the first time and driving home. Nothing. (Except maybe cutting their fingernails for the first time.)

Heading home with your baby is such a momentous occasion—for me, it felt like we were truly a family when we were all home together. And while the first few weeks (or even months) at home can be tricky, they're also lovely in their own way. Enjoy this time, and don't expect too much of yourself—or your baby. Ignore everyone who asks how the baby is sleeping. Ignore everyone who tells you to sleep while the baby is sleeping (I don't know a single woman who is able to do this). Be kind to yourself, let others help, and if they don't offer, tell people what you need.

Oh, and take lots of pics—these first few weeks feel like an eternity, but believe me, they just fly right by.

Home time

Routines

· · · · · · · · · ·

When I was pregnant with Oscar, I imagined that I'd go back to work pretty quickly. We were adamant—like most first-time parents—that we wouldn't be those 'routine' parents. We'd go with the flow, the baby would fit in around us. Ha! We pretty quickly figured out that that wasn't reasonable. In fact, when we first had Oscar, we were both so shell-shocked by the ways our lives had changed, I remember looking at Chris one day and saying, 'Why did we do this? I don't want this baby anymore, do you?' He said, 'I can't believe people go back for more. Why?' We were in shock for a long time. Oscar had reflux and didn't sleep at all at night. He would sleep *alllll* day . . . and then party once the sun went down. It was a huge shift for me; I was used to being in complete control—I'm the girl with the totally organised diary—and suddenly, I had this baby who just would not cooperate. I kept thinking, 'What have I done to my life?' It was not at all what I expected it to be.

One of the lowest points came when we were still in the hospital. Chris had a game and so my sister was with me, but Oscar was crying and would not calm down. He didn't want to be fed, he didn't want to be rocked, nothing was working to help him. I felt totally defeated and I'd barely even begun! I kept thinking, *I am not cut out for this. I can't do this.* I was bawling. Finally a midwife came in and said, 'Would you like me to take him?' And I thought, *How long can you keep him for?*

Around the six-week mark, I called on a paediatric sleep consultant to come and help. I was at my wit's end. There is a reason they use sleep deprivation to torture people: because it bloody works. I was exhausted. Oscar was unhappy. I was so unhappy.

I didn't even know sleep consultants existed before Oscar was born—but thank god they do! Naively, I assumed that babies slept like . . . well, babies. (Seriously, where does the saying 'sleep like a baby' come from?)

The sleep consultant turned out to be a bloody miracle worker. She said to me, 'You go to sleep, I'll sort him out.' So I did. I went to bed at 7.30 that night and woke up at 7 the next morning. When I woke up, I thought, 'Oh my god, what's going on? Where is he? What's happened?' But I went downstairs

Awake time

Babies can get overstimulated and overtired very easily. Babies under three months will have very little awake time between naps. Between three and six months, your baby will be awake from 1.5 to 3 hours between naps. From six to twelve months, this will increase to 2–3 hours of awake time.

and found Oscar sitting in his rocker, happy as a clam. It was amazing. Within six weeks, he was sleeping from 7 p.m. to 7 a.m. every night.

My sleep consultant taught me the importance of routine and identifying sleep cues. Babies need sleep, but they aren't always great at knowing when and how to get themselves to sleep. That's where we, as parents, can step in and help them. I really believe helping your babies settle into a good routine is one of the greatest gifts you can give them.

Why I love routines

I am a routine mum through and through. I'm a strong believer that babies will begin to sleep through the night sooner if they are in a routine. (But some babies just do it naturally on their own from very early on—how lucky for their mamas.) Humans in general, I believe, thrive on routine. Personally, I take great comfort in knowing not only how my days are planned out, but also my weeks. Routines allow me to plan and look forward to things. For example, every single morning, I know I wake up at 7 a.m. and so do my kids. We come downstairs, put the coffee machine on, I change the twins' nappies, and make breakfast for Oscar and Billie. By then, the coffee machine has heated up and I'll make myself a strong latte and sip it as I feed the twins. There's a lot going on, but we all know what's supposed to be happening, which makes everything run a lot smoother.

I am flexible with my routines—if I have a day where nap times go out the window, I know it's not the end of the world. The beauty of a routine is that you can slip back into it easily the next day. There are times when Chris and I get so busy with work that we simply can't stick to the routine, and no doubt, this will happen to you at some point, too. When we're on a routine, everyone sleeps better (and for longer!), so I really dread those times when we let go of the routine. My kids seem to crave routine and so do I.

Routines aren't for everyone and you need to decide what suits your family and lifestyle. Personally, routines have helped me go back to work, allowed my husband to work (and train, when he was playing footy), and most importantly, kept us happy and sane. Routines also help when other people— like grandparents and babysitters, or later, daycare educators—are looking after your children. It's so much easier to say to someone who's caring for your kids, 'They have lunch at 11, a nap at 12, and should be up by about 2.30.'

When to start the routine

While newborn babies can be difficult to put on a routine, it's important to start a 'wake-eat-play-sleep' routine early on. Oscar started sleeping through the night (7 p.m.–7 a.m.) at twelve weeks, and Billie started sleeping through at six weeks (with a dream feed). The key difference? I started Oscar on a routine when he was six weeks old and it took six weeks to 'kick in'. With Billie, I started her routine as soon as she was born. So the earlier you can implement a routine, the better it will be for everyone.

Identifying sleep cues

I cannot stress how important it is to be able to detect sleep signs in your little one. If you miss the boat with these (like we did with Oscar for so many weeks), it makes it much harder for your baby to fall asleep as they are overtired. (You know how you feel when you're overtired? Try being a baby, who can only communicate by crying.) I remember having Oscar up for four hours at a time as a five-week-old—which is just crazy, looking back. But to me, at that stage, he didn't seem tired at all. He had these big, wide-open eyes—how could he need a nap? Turns out, those big wide eyes were actually bug eyes—he was exhausted!

These are the sleep cues to look out for:

* yawning (duh, I know)
* staring into space (or even going cross-eyed)
* red-rimmed eyes
* irritability
* pulling on ears
* closing fists
* arching backwards, or making jerky movements
* sucking on fingers.

Buy a notebook

You don't need fancy equipment or even an app to start a routine. I suggest buying a notebook (just an ordinary notebook!) so you can write down what is happening in your child's day, like when they wake, feed and sleep. Keeping track of these things will show you a pattern. (And in those first few weeks, you're probably so tired and overwhelmed that you won't be able to remember exactly when your baby woke, fed, which breast they fed from and so on. Writing it down takes the pressure off.) Writing down your baby's activities provides a guide as to what is to come next and also allows you to problem-solve. Why do they get grizzly around 4 p.m.? Have they been awake too long? Do they sleep better at night when they've had an extra nap during the day?

Routine One: Newborns

Look, newborns are so bloody hard to put on a routine—perhaps even impossible. (You know what? I don't even know if I should use the words 'newborn' and 'routine' in the same sentence.) Newborns are very sleepy, and need to feed a lot. It can be really stressful to try to keep up a schedule with a newborn—I know my babies loved to 'suck and snooze' (i.e. feed and then immediately fall asleep on the boob). This was really frustrating—I was anxious that they weren't feeding enough, or learning how to 'sleep properly'. I've since learned that, as a mum to a newborn, you have so much to worry about—try not to let strict routines be one of them. Setting up a rough routine is great, but it doesn't need to be anything concrete right now. If you can get your baby on a basic routine, you're setting them up to be able to transition into a more structured one once they become more alert and can sustain longer awake times.

GENERAL RULES

* Feed every 3–4 hours. Wake them if they are still sleeping (which is most of the time)—yes, even overnight. The aim is to encourage your baby to gain as much weight as possible so they are big enough to sustain longer periods of sleep overnight. Short-term pain, long-term gain, as they say.
* Always swaddle tightly and safely.
* During the day, it's OK to go with the flow and follow your baby's lead a little more. But night-time routines are very important—they help your baby differentiate night from day, and start to associate night with sleeping, and day with waking.
* 7 p.m. is bedtime. You might want to do a bath at 6.30, followed by a feed, and then bed. You don't have to do this, but a bath can help calm your baby and help them associate bath time with bedtime shortly after.
* If it suits your family, do Midwife Cath's routine of the bath at 10 p.m., and let your partner take the reins. This way, you can get some extra sleep and your partner can get some bonding time in. We did this with Oscar for about the first ten weeks, and it worked really well.

* Set your alarm for 2 a.m., and wake your baby for a feed. I know, it seems absurd: wake a sleeping baby? Are you crazy, Judd? I know, I know. But believe me, a baby who is well fed will gain weight more quickly, be more settled, and be ready to drop this overnight feed earlier.
* Wake up for the day between 6 and 7 a.m. If your baby wakes before 6, give a small feed, and then a larger one at 7 a.m., to reinforce that this is the true start of the day.

Routine Two: 4–6 weeks

At around four weeks, your baby will need more awake time, and less time napping. This can be hard—babies at this age still want to sleep a lot during the day, but this can really mess with their night-time sleeping. Try to start a 'feed-play-sleep' routine, where your baby is awake for about 1–1.5 hours between each nap. This will ensure they get enough sleep so that they're not overtired, but also that they don't get too much sleep and won't settle for you at night.

7 a.m.	wake and feed
8–10 a.m.	nap
10 a.m.	wake and feed
12–2 p.m.	nap
2 p.m.	wake and feed
4–5 p.m.	nap
6 p.m.	bath, followed by feed
7 p.m.	sleep
11 p.m.	wake and feed, then put straight back down to bed
3 a.m.	set alarm, wake and feed

Routine Three: 6–12 weeks

At six weeks, your baby will probably have gained enough weight for you to start thinking about dropping their overnight feed. At this stage, Billie was over 5 kilograms, so I was comfortable with not feeding her overnight. Initially, she'd sometimes wake around 4.30 a.m. In this instance, I'd feed her a small amount to get her through, and then wake her again at 7 a.m. to start the day. Sometimes she would stir at around 5 a.m., but I would leave her if she was only fussing, not crying. After a moment, she'd put herself back to sleep, and sleep again till 7 a.m.

7 a.m.	wake and feed
8–10 a.m.	nap
10 a.m.	wake and feed
12–2 p.m.	nap
2 p.m.	wake and feed
4–5 p.m.	nap
6 p.m.	bath, followed by feed
7 p.m.	sleep
11 p.m.	wake and feed, then put straight back down to bed

Routine Four: 3–4 months

At this stage, you can drop the 'dream feed' (i.e. the 11 p.m. feed)—you just make up for it with an extra feed during the day.

7 a.m.	wake and feed
8.30–11 a.m.	nap
11 a.m.	wake and feed
12.30–3 p.m.	nap
3 p.m.	wake and feed
4 p.m.	nap (no longer than 40 minutes)
6 p.m.	bath
6.30 p.m.	feed
7 p.m.	sleep

Routine Five: 4–6 months

At this point, your baby will need more awake time during the day. Use this time to get out into the sunshine, read books with your baby and start playing with them. They'll be so much more responsive by this stage, which is just so lovely. Enjoy it!

7 a.m.	wake and feed
9–11 a.m.	nap
11 a.m.	wake and feed
1–3 p.m.	nap
3 p.m.	wake and feed
4.30 p.m.	nap (no longer than twenty minutes)
6 p.m.	bath
6.30 p.m.	feed
7 p.m.	sleep

Every baby is different

While I have followed the above routines with great success, keep in mind that every baby is different (and I'm no sleep expert)—this is just a rough guide of what I do based on the professional advice I sought. If you have a baby who struggles to sleep and it's causing a lot of grief (and believe me, I get it), then I would consider seeking professional advice. I am a *huge* advocate of seeking help when you need it; there are no medals for doing this on your own, and raising your hand is not a sign of weakness or defeat. Babies are bloody hard and as they say, it takes a village to raise one. Sometimes that village will include a sleep consultant. And trust me: when your baby starts to sleep, you will start to sleep, too. And everything—and I mean everything—will be better.

Routine Six: The twins

As we've established, I'm a routine mum. But that said, all four of my babies have had slightly different routines. They're all variations on the same theme, but being flexible *within a routine* allowed me to set a great schedule for each of my babies, at each stage of their—and our—lives. With Oscar, for instance, we only had to worry about one baby, so following a very strict routine was easy, and doing certain things at certain times of the day wasn't a problem. For example, Chris would bath Oscar at 10 p.m. when he was really little. At the time, it suited us. (Meaning: it allowed me to go to bed after his 6 p.m. feed!) Chris would get Oscar up around 10 p.m., give him a bath and a bottle and pop him to bed around 11 p.m. This meant that I didn't have to get up to feed Oscar until around 2 a.m., by which time I'd had hours of sleep and wasn't feeling as foul as one would usually expect at 2 a.m.

With Billie, the late bath didn't really suit us. After chasing Oscar, who was then a toddler, around all day, nobody wanted to get the baby up at 10 p.m.—we were all exhausted. So we stuck to the 6 p.m. bath for her and that worked perfectly for our family at that time in our lives.

The twins were a slightly different story again. Placed on a four-hour routine with military precision by the special care nursery midwives (AKA Angels Sent Directly From Heaven) at Frances Perry House, Tom and Darcy were whipped into a *perfect* routine from day one. And look, if 35-week premmies can be placed on a routine at one day old, then *anyone* can.

Here's what the twins' routine looked like at the newborn stage:

6 a.m.	wake, nappy change, feed, sleep
10 a.m.	wake, nappy change, feed, sleep
2 p.m.	wake, nappy change, feed, sleep
5.30 p.m.	wake and bath
6 p.m.	feed, sleep
10 p.m.	wake, nappy change, feed, sleep
2 a.m.	wake, nappy change, feed, sleep

The boys were bottle-fed which made this routine very easy to implement as I had set volumes of milk they had to take at each feed as prescribed by their paediatrician. I wouldn't stop the feed until they'd finished their bottle and I think, because they were so well fed, it made them stick to their routine very easily.

Once they reached their target weight we dropped the 2 a.m. feed and made sure they had bigger feeds for the remaining five bottle feeds so as to meet the paediatrician's quota. Once they met their next target weight we dropped the 10 p.m. 'dream feed' and again, upped their intake for their remaining four bottle feeds to meet the quota. Talk to your healthcare professional about how many millilitres per day your baby should be getting and this will guide your feeding routine.

The bottom line

So there you have it. Six slightly different routines—but all with the same basics. Choose one (or none) that works for your family and use these routines as a guide to shape your own. You will find you have variations that will suit your baby and your lifestyle. And please, don't get too caught up trying to stick exactly to one of my baby's routines. The last thing I want you to think is, *Gah, Bec Bloody Judd's babies were feeding at 6 p.m. but mine won't feed until 6.30. WHAT HAVE I DONE WRONG?* The short answer is, you've done nothing wrong. Let these routines be a guide, but figure out what is best for you and your family. You'll get there. If I can, anyone can!

Interruption from an expert

Why you should wrap your baby

Here's Midwife Cath on the importance of swaddling your baby in their first few months. I know, I know—it seems like a hassle when you've already got so much to do. But trust me, swaddling makes a big difference to your newborn's sleep.

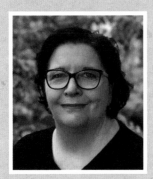

The Midwife
Cathryn Curtin

Why is it important to wrap your baby?

I am a big advocate of wrapping babies. When your baby was in your uterus, they were safe and very comfortable. When your baby moved within the uterus, they would feel resistance from the surrounding walls—so even when moving about, the baby felt contained and safe.

Babies are born with primitive reflexes that are hardwired into their brains as survival methods. These reflexes help keep your baby alive. The most prominent reflexes are the Moro reflex, crying and the sucking reflex. These reflexes allow your newborn baby to communicate with you—to tell you that they are hot, cold or hungry.

What is the Moro reflex?

The Moro reflex is a primitive reflex that helps your baby feel safe. Picture your baby on a change table, or in a cot: when your baby cries, the arms stretch out, looking for comfort. When your baby was in the uterus, the confines of the space provided that. By wrapping your baby, you'll give your baby the comfort and security babies crave. Your baby will sleep better and feel more at ease in the world.

So why are people worried about wrapping?

There are some legitimate concerns about wrapping, and chief among them is that wrapping too tightly can cause damage to the hips. I have invented a wrapping technique (see my app, Cath's Wrap) that negates this problem. You can also buy zip-up swaddles that keep your baby wrapped without being too tight.

How long do I need to wrap my baby for?

I suggest wrapping your baby for the first 6–8 weeks during the day, but at night I wrap for up to six months, unless they are starting to roll. As your baby grows and becomes more stable with the Moro reflex, you won't need to wrap as much during the day. By six months, you won't need to wrap your baby for sleeping— you can safely transfer your baby to a sleeping bag.

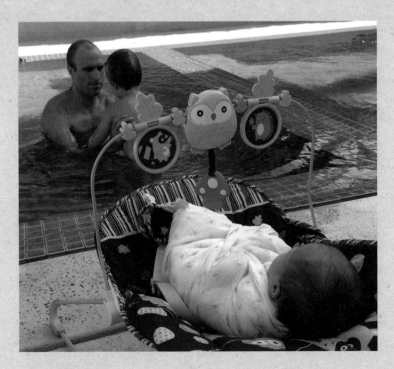

All wrapped up!

Sleeping FAQs

After having Oscar and realising that I had no freaking idea (to say the very least) how to get babies (especially my own) to sleep . . . but also, that there are actually professionally trained people out there who do just that, I didn't dillydally with Billie and made sure I enlisted help from Tahna Leader, the woman who helped me get Oscar sleeping well. She put Billie on an amazing routine which I followed to a tee and whammo, Billie first slept through at four weeks. *True story.* Then, from six weeks, she slept through every single night. What an angel. Tahna, I mean. Billie's quite sweet, too.

With the twins, I knew there was no time for mucking around, so I enlisted paediatric sleep consultant Amanda McGill. Amanda trained with Tahna so she followed the same sleep science theories, and came highly recommended by many friends and family members who had used her with a 100 per cent success rate. Knowing I had her to help me when the twins came helped to alleviate some of the anxiety I was feeling about having two newborns at once. Amanda's evidence-based approach really suited the science nerd in me; I liked seeing the methodology to her practice. It really was a matter of balancing the calories my babies needed, along with specific sleep and awake times during the day. As the routine worked so well I've never had to do the whole cry-it-out thing. My babies usually went to sleep quite easily because they had full tummies and were ready for bed—the routine made sure of that. Sure, I would let them grizzle every now and again when I put them down (this is a normal part of a baby settling itself to sleep), but I never had to resort to letting my babies cry for extended periods; I wouldn't be comfortable doing that, anyway. Both Tahna and Amanda taught me the difference between an 'I'm putting myself to sleep' grizzle (which to the new mother of a firstborn can sound like the child is screaming bloody murder!) and a proper emotional cry, which needs to be attended to straight away.

Amanda prescribed a wonderful routine for my premmie twins that flowed on perfectly from the four-hourly feed routine they were placed on in hospital. We continued this and then, as they grew and developed, Amanda guided me by adapting their routine along the way. We (ahem, she!) had them sleeping through very early on indeed. They were thriving, happy and, to this day, have been perfect sleepers.

Interruption from an expert

Newborn routines

Paediatric sleep expert Amanda McGill explains the ins and outs of newborn routines.

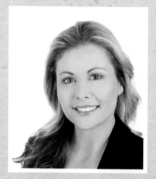

The Paediatric Sleep Expert
Amanda McGill

Why should I follow a routine with my baby?

Humans are diurnal—that is, active by day, inactive at night. This behaviour is regulated by our built-in body clock (known as the circadian rhythm) that responds primarily to light (day) and darkness (night). We also each have a set amount of 'wake versus sleep' time we require to function and learn. By following a routine, we aim to maintain this equilibrium. So yes, even if you think you don't follow a routine yourself, you do, even if it is as simple as 'be awake during the day, sleep during the night'.

For babies, following a flexible routine from birth has many benefits. Not only does it support their body clock as it starts to mature, but it also gets them into good habits early by making sure they feed, play and sleep when needed. This helps the days to become more predictable for both you and your baby. We all thrive on routine, and sleep and eat so much better when a habitual daily routine is established.

When should I start a routine with my baby?

I recommend all parents follow a flexible routine from birth. By flexible routine, I mean a combination of baby-led and parent-led factors.

Newborns have immature eating and sleeping patterns and as such, they feed and sleep best on demand. However, because they also have no concept of day or night, they do need some structure put in place to help guide them in the right direction. Without parent-led structure, babies can get their days and nights mixed up, or they may not eat enough. By keeping daytimes bright and active, revolving around feed, play, sleep and settle cycles, and keeping night-times dark and inactive as far as feed, sleep and settle cycles go, you will help your baby quickly learn to be active in the day and inactive at night—and therefore, sleep through the night faster.

However, learning to feed, play, sleep and settle isn't smooth sailing for newborns. That's why a flexible routine is important. Once sleep patterns begin to mature (from week 6) and effective feeding is mastered (that is, the ability to take a full feed and regularly gain weight), a stricter, more time-based routine can be followed (this usually occurs by about two to three months).

What does a routine look like for a new baby?

Newborns generally cycle through the day in a feed, play, sleep, settle pattern that runs over 2–4 hours. The following is an example of a baby who feeds every four hours, and can stay awake for approximately 1 hour.

7 a.m.

Eat: Wake baby and feed. Feed your baby as much as they want. (Note: it can take some newborns a good 40–60 minutes to feed well. Be patient!)

Once finished, burp well. (Newborns have immature digestive systems and require help to be burped.)

Change nappy.

Play: Go for a walk, read your baby a book, engage in floor play or tummy time.

8 a.m.

Sleep: Prepare baby for bed once tired/sleepy (for example, wrap in a swaddle and take them to their room). Settle baby to sleep.

Settle: Settle/resettle baby on and off until next feed time.

11 a.m.

Eat: Wake baby and feed. Once finished, burp well. Change nappy.

Play: Go for a walk, read your baby a book, engage in floor play or tummy time.

12 p.m.

Sleep: Prepare baby for bed once tired/sleepy. Settle baby to sleep.

Settle: Settle/resettle baby on and off until next feed time.

3 p.m.

Eat: Wake baby and feed. Once finished, burp well. Change nappy.

Play: Go for a walk, read your baby a book, engage in floor play or tummy time.

4 p.m.

Nap: Prepare baby for bed once tired/sleepy. Settle baby to sleep. For this nap, do not allow baby to sleep more than 80 minutes, as this could interfere with night sleeping.

Settle: Settle/resettle baby on and off until next feed time.

5.30 p.m.

Eat: Wake baby and feed (this may only be a half feed at this stage, as you'll feed again soon).

6.15 p.m.

Play: Bedtime routine (bath, quiet play).

6.30–7 p.m.

Sleep/eat: Prepare baby for bed. Offer baby a top-up feed then settle baby to sleep.

Settle: Settle/resettle baby on and off until next feed time.

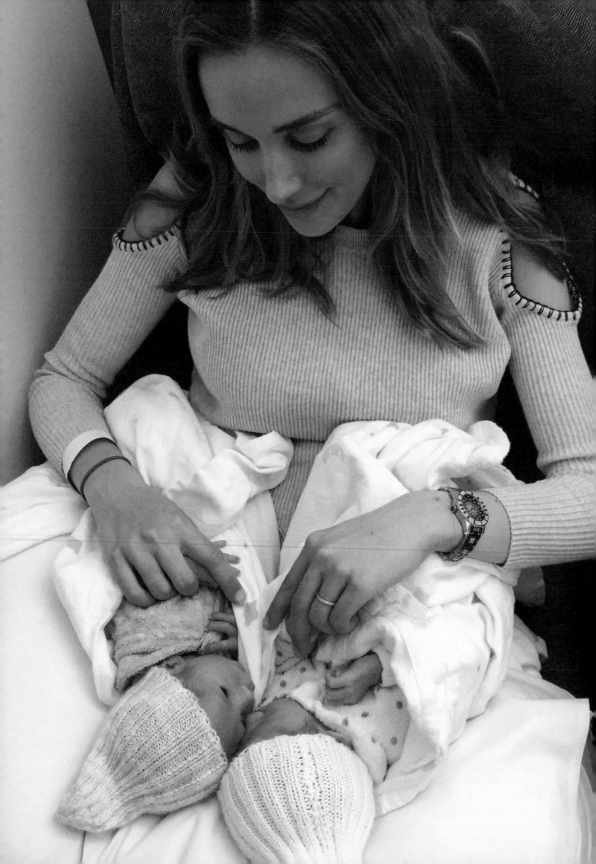

11 p.m.

    Eat/sleep: Wake baby and feed (this is called a 'dream feed') then settle back to sleep.

    Settle: Settle/resettle baby on and off until next feed time.

3 a.m.

    Eat/sleep: Wake baby and feed then settle back to sleep. Note: if baby is gaining weight well they can also be left to self-wake here and feed on demand, rather than you waking them.

    Settle: Settle/resettle baby on and off until next feed time.

7 a.m.

    Time to start the day again!

What are the most important things I need to think about when implementing a routine?

There are lots of things to consider: when do you want to start and end the day? What things would you like to incorporate into your baby's ritual? (For example, is a daily bath important? Would you like to do one of your baby's naps as a pram walk?)

However, I think flexibility is probably the most important factor. While routines are important and give much-needed structure to family life, your family's current dynamics and your baby's natural rhythm and routine may not always align. This is perfectly normal and OK. Keep in mind that the day will always be a bit of give and take between parent-led and baby-led activities. (Hey, welcome to parenthood!)

What things might interrupt or impede a routine?

Unrealistic expectations and a lack of consistency will impede a routine.

To avoid this, ensure your expectations for your baby's eat-play-sleep needs are appropriate. Some babies eat best every two hours, some do best every three hours, others can hold out for four. For many parents, it's a matter of trial and error: go with your baby's natural flow and see what works. The same goes for sleep requirements. Some babies need lots of sleep, others not as much. Forcing babies to eat and/or sleep when they are not ready can cause the eat-play-sleep cycle to become out of balance, which can then lead to a very unsettled baby and a routine that goes out the window.

Consistency with eat-play-sleep rituals is also important. A lack of consistency—for instance, settling your baby for a nap at 9 a.m. one day, but waiting until 11 a.m. the next—can send mixed signals to your baby and confuse them.

How early can a baby sleep through the night?

The million-dollar question!

Babies primarily wake at night to eat because they have small tummies but high caloric needs. Over time, a baby will learn to eat more and stretch their tummies, enabling them to go longer between feeds. Most babies will begin to sleep through when they can eat all their calories in the day. This is typically around three to four months. Some babies can sleep through as early as four weeks, but others will take six months (this may be with or without a dream feed). It takes time, and sleeping through the night is about your baby's needs. Try not to compare your baby with others in this regard.

What is a dream feed? When do I start this? When do I drop it?

A dream feed is when a baby is woken in the late evening and offered a feed around the time the parent wants to go to bed (normally between 9 and 11 p.m.). After feeding, babies can sleep for several hours, so waking baby to feed can ensure the parent gets a few hours of unbroken sleep. Dream feeds can be started from birth and are usually dropped once baby is feeding well in the day (any time between three and six months).

Keep in mind that some babies don't feed well when woken, so this won't work for all babies. Some may be best to feed on demand overnight instead. It's an experiment.

I've heard you should never wake a sleeping baby—is that true?

No! It can take babies a few months to develop their own circadian rhythm (that day/night pattern we talked about earlier), and they have small tummies but high caloric needs. They must therefore learn to eat well and regularly in the day/evening and should be woken to do so. If babies are not woken to feed at least once every four hours, they will more often than not demand extra feeds.

And, on the other hand, it's also important to encourage awake periods in the day to help regulate your baby's circadian rhythms further. This can be difficult with a newborn—they seem to always want to sleep—but eventually you'll be able to stretch out your baby's awake time effectively.

How do poor sleeping habits develop?

In my experience, lack of routine and understanding that self-settling is important are the two biggest culprits.

Our day must be filled with a balance of eat, play and sleep. Without a routine, it's hard to know if the baby's needs for each of these are being met. Babies don't sleep well, or for very long, if they are hungry. They can also get overtired very easily if they are awake for too long.

It's also important to know that babies cry when they are tired—it is their only way of communicating, and though none of us want to hear our little ones in distress, crying is a normal part of self-settling. Forming sleep associations—like rocking, dummy use and feeding to sleep—can cause your baby to be a dependent sleeper who always needs assistance, even years down the track.

Following a routine eat-play-sleep cycle where baby has all its needs met encourages self-settling and the development of independent sleep skills. While it is OK to help newborns fall asleep, there comes a time when they are ready to learn how to self-settle—for most babies, this is around six weeks. Sleep is a skill that needs to be taught, but it is also a transitional process, which takes time. Be patient. With consistency, it will happen.

My baby will only fall asleep when fed to sleep. What do I do?

With newborns, this is OK—very young babies are generally very sleepy and find it difficult to stay awake long enough to feed properly.

However, if you make this a habit, feeding to sleep can be a very hard association to break. Aim to follow a feed-play-sleep-settle routine during the day where possible. Ensure baby is feeding well (taking as much as they need) at feed time. A dummy can also be a good way to get a baby to settle without a feed; once they are able to settle without the feed the dummy can be eliminated. If baby still insists on feeding before sleep, aim to feed baby then rouse them after the feed so they don't fall completely asleep (we want to wake them up just enough to know they have stopped feeding). Babies remember what they were doing when they fall asleep so when they wake, will often want that memory back. If they fall asleep while you are rocking them, for instance, they expect you to be rocking them when they wake again. By waking them up after the feed, their last memory isn't then of feeding but of lying awake in their cot.

My baby wants to stay up and party after the 2 a.m. feed. How do I get my baby to fall straight back asleep and differentiate day from night?

* During the evening, use only the dimmest of lights (or none at all, if possible). Exposure to bright, artificial lighting in the evening can cause us to wake up, making it harder to fall back asleep.

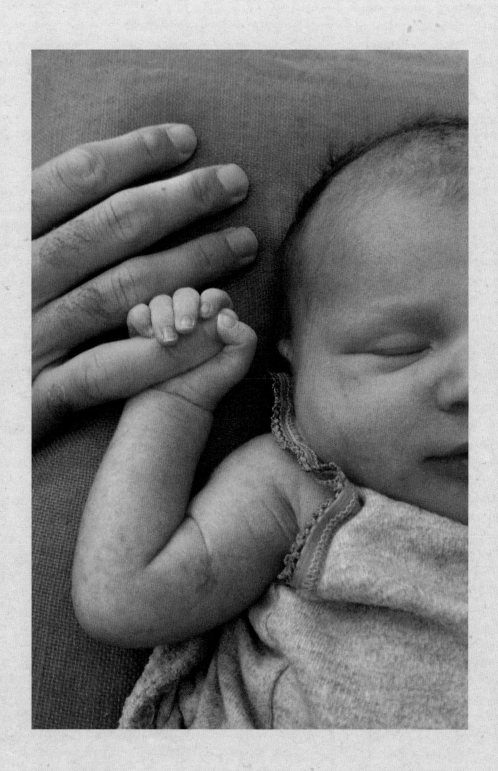

* Keep night feeds dull, dark and boring. No talking, no playing, minimal eye contact.
* Change your baby's nappy only if necessary. Changing can help wake your baby up (which will encourage them to have a full feed), but it can wake them up *too* much; avoid changing them if you can.
* Ensure your baby has plenty of active awake periods in the day. I find getting out and about—going for a walk, getting a coffee, doing the groceries—can really help with this.
* Keep playtimes bright and sunny in the day.
* If you follow these tips, babies will usually learn that night-time is for sleeping and settle back to sleep after night feeds pretty quickly.

My baby falls asleep before taking a full feed. How do I keep them awake?

Newborns aren't able to stay awake for long—at most, 90 minutes at a time. It's therefore common for them to get sleepy or fall asleep while feeding, especially if they take more than 30 minutes to feed.

To keep your baby awake long enough to have a full feed, try the following:
* Follow a feed-play-sleep cycle. By feeding as soon as they wake, babies will have energy to feed effectively. If feeds are delayed too long, baby can become too tired to feed properly and will fall asleep while feeding.
* Keep your baby cool. Unwrap your baby and expose some skin, perhaps removing their legs or feet from their suit. Awake time is active time for babies and feeding is like a workout. If your baby is too warm, they will fall asleep.
* Keep your baby active. Interact with them. Tickle them. Talk to them. Read. Head out of the house. Turn the radio on.
* Take a break and do something active for a few minutes, for

example, change their nappy, or put them on a play mat. Then try feeding them again.

Each baby has a different feeding style. Babies usually alternate between one of four feeding styles, which are:

1. Feeds all in one go.

2. Has a three-quarter feed, stops for a break, then has the last quarter.

3. Has half a feed, stops for a break, then has the last half.

4. Has a quarter feed, stops for a break, then has the last three-quarters.

Tip: Always attempt to offer feeds on and off a few times until you think the feed is finished. Allow 40–60 minutes for each feed, to ensure enough time for your baby to take a full feed. It is common for newborns to need the occasional break when feeding. Feeding is hard work and can make them tired.

My baby always wakes after 40 minutes. How do I stretch sleeps out?

Babies, like adults, sleep in cycles. Unlike adults, babies have relatively short sleep cycles of 40 minutes.

Newborns need lots of sleep so should generally sleep for longer than 40 minutes after a full feed. If your baby wakes at around 40 minutes, they should be resettled until their next approximate feed time. Patting, rocking, a cuddle, a dummy and/or wearing the baby in a carrier can help them go back to sleep and stretch out the next feed time. A feed or top-up can also be offered if your baby didn't eat enough at the last feed.

From six weeks, sleep patterns begin maturing and babies should be settled and resettled to sleep in their cots from an awake-but-drowsy state, with minimal aids to avoid sleep associations developing. Rhythmically patting baby intermittently on their tummy when in their cot can help them settle/resettle back to sleep quite easily. White noise can also help.

Is it OK to let a newborn cry to sleep?

No. Newborns should be settled to sleep and resettled when necessary, as their sleep patterns are immature. From six to eight weeks, when sleep patterns begin to mature, infants can gently be taught to self-settle but this should still be done with assistance (for instance, by using the tummy-patting technique described above).

Do I need to wrap my baby for sleep?

No, but I strongly recommend that you do. Wrapping can help babies sleep for longer stretches between feeds and at night, compared with unwrapped infants.

Babies have strong rooting and startle reflexes that can wake them from sleep. The rooting reflex is triggered when their mouth or lips are touched, causing them to begin suckling. The startle reflex (Moro reflex) causes involuntary arm jerking in response to noises and/or a sense of no support. When babies are wrapped with their hands away from their face, they feel more secure. It limits activation of these reflexes, allowing them to sleep longer and through sleep cycles.

These reflexes diminish as babies get older (this can be any time from two to four months). Once diminished, wrapping should stop so babies can learn to sleep with their arms free and use their hands and fingers to self-soothe if needed. Wrapping for too long (over four to six months) can lead to an inability to self-settle. Wrapping should also cease once babies show signs of learning to roll (around four to six months), to enable them to learn to roll around in their sleep safely.

I'm sticking to the routine, but my baby is still unsettled. Why?

Unfortunately, babies can cry a lot. The good thing is that crying is usually a sign of normal, healthy infant development. Bear in mind that infants up to six weeks cry an average of three hours a day.

As many as one in five parents report concerns with their infants' crying and unsettledness. It can be very stressful not to know why your baby is crying or unsettled. It's important to know that babies cry for many different reasons, most of which you'll learn as you get to know your baby.

A great way to try to understand some of the common reasons why your baby could be crying and unsettled is to learn the Dunstan Baby Language system. This is based on decoding pre-emptive sounds made pre-crying and is based on reflexes. These include:

* sucking reflex: 'Neh'—I am hungry/want to suckle
* tired reflex: 'Owh'—I am sleepy
* wind reflex: 'Eh'—I need to burp
* gas reflex: 'Eairh'—I have gas pains
* uncomfortable reflex: 'Heh'—I am uncomfortable (too hot/ cold/itchy).

Other causes of excessive crying can include:

* overstimulation (when your baby has been awake too long and/or been exposed to too much activity)
* reflux
* other medical/dietary issues (eczema, allergies, intolerances, etc.).

Many infants become quite settled and cry less once:

* their sleep patterns start maturing (between six to eight weeks)
* their feeding habits improve
* they begin to follow a predictable daily routine.

If in doubt about your baby's crying/unsettledness, always seek medical advice, especially if they cry for more than three hours a day.

Seeking help

When it comes to sleep, it's so important to seek help if things aren't going well. Sleep deprivation is a horrible, horrible thing—for both you and your baby. And while it's not reasonable for everyone to have a sleep consultant come to their home, the good news is that there are plenty of accessible options out there. Your first port of call should always be your GP, who can recommend local services. Then, depending on where you live, there's MotherCare, Tresilian, Karitane and more.

For a list of sleep help in your state, head to **m.raisingchildren.net.au**. Most of these services are covered by Medicare.

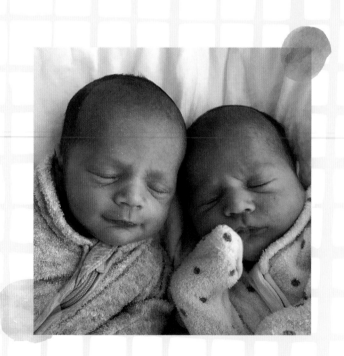

Darcy and Tom

Safe sleeping tips

Bringing home a new baby is exhilarating—and completely terrifying. When you're in the hospital, everything is so calm and ordered. Your baby looks so content and safe in their clear plastic bassinet. If the shit hits the fan, at least you're in hospital, and you can get help literally by clicking a button. Huge relief, right?

Once you get home, though, and place your baby in their bassinet or cot to sleep, you will think about the heartbreaking possibility of sudden infant death syndrome (SIDS). Like any new parent, I would stress out every time I put Oscar down for a nap, wondering what would happen if he wiggled free of his swaddle or blanket, or what if he magically learned to roll over during an REM cycle? As he got older, my worries began to dissipate, but even now when I think back on those early days, I remember how I prayed he would stay safe all night. With that in mind, here are the current recommendations for safe sleeping.

SIDS and SUDI

* Sudden infant death syndrome (also known as cot death, or crib death) occurs in babies aged less than one year (and most commonly, between one and four months). No one is quite sure what exactly causes SIDS, but it occurs when babies are asleep.
* Sudden unexplained death in infancy is the term used to refer to both SIDS and other fatal sleep accidents, like unintentional suffocation.

What does a safe sleeping space look like?

A safe sleeping environment is one where all potential dangers have been removed.

* Babies should sleep in a cot.
* Babies should sleep on a firm, flat mattress that meets Australian safety standards.
* The cot should be fitted with safe bedding. Safe bedding is tucked in firmly, without a pillow or blankets that can accidentally cover a baby's head.
* Babies should sleep in this cot both during the night and day.

Never let your baby sleep . . .

. . . unattended on an adult bed or bunk bed, on a waterbed, beanbag, couch, pillow or cushion, or with a sleeping adult or child on a couch, sofa or chair.

Watch out for cot surroundings

Where is your baby's cot? Have a look at the space around it. Are there hanging cords (such as those attached to blinds, curtains or electrical appliances) that could get caught around your baby's neck? Time to move the cot. Also, keep heaters (or any electrical appliances, really) well away from the cot to avoid the risk of overheating, burns and electrocution.

Heat and SIDS

Overheating has been shown to be a contributing factor to SIDS. Never use electric blankets, hot water bottles or wheat bags for babies. Dress your baby for bed as you would yourself—not too hot, not too cold. Layers—like a singlet and a onesie—work well. Never cover your baby's head with a beanie or hat while they are sleeping.

Use a sleeping bag

While I'm a big fan of swaddling early on, as your baby gets older (around three to six months), using a sleeping bag is a great idea. A properly fitted sleeping bag (with a fitted neck, no hood, and of course, one that is the right size for your baby) will reduce the risk of bedclothes (like sheets and blankets) covering your baby's face (you won't need them), and can also delay rolling until your baby has passed the peak age of SUDI by promoting back sleep. They also help to keep your baby's temperature at a more constant level.

What goes in the cot

The baby. That's about it, really. Put your baby in a fitted sleeping bag or swaddle, and place them in the cot. You can use a blanket, but only if it is snugly tucked into the sides of the cot, and not near your baby's face. Soft bedding (like pillows, quilts, doonas, soft toys and bumpers) are dangerous and shouldn't be used.

The best sleeping position

Your baby should be placed *on their back* at the bottom of the cot, with their feet touching the end (this will ensure baby doesn't move down any further, potentially going under a sheet). Make sure if a blanket is used it only reaches their chest.

What about co-sleeping?

While I know co-sleeping is popular, the research shows that sharing a sleep surface with your baby increases the risk of SUDI and SIDS (particularly for babies who are less than three months old, premature or small for their age).

The risks of co-sleeping are even greater if parents have been smoking, drinking or taking drugs.

Remember that co-sleeping is not just about sharing a bed—there's a very high risk of SUDI and SIDS when babies share a couch with an adult during sleep.

What about twins?

Just like single babies, the safest way to sleep twins is in their own safe sleeping container (i.e. cot, bassinette or cradle) in your room for the first six to twelve months (although all of my babies slept in their own cots, in their own rooms, from day one).

Some parents put twins in the same cot, to sleep together, but this can be dangerous—what if one twin were to accidentally cover the face of the other, for example?

If you're travelling or absolutely must put your twins in the same cot, don't let them share bedding, and place them at opposite ends of the cot.

Why share a room?

While not everyone will place their baby's cot in their own room, SIDS guidelines state that doing so reduces the risk of SIDS, SUDI and fatal sleep accidents during both day naps and night-time sleeps. It's recommended you keep your baby's cot in your room for the first six to twelve months.

Baby gear: The stuff you'll need later

For such a small person, your baby sure has a lot of stuff. And trust me, their stuff just grows and grows . . . and grows. While you don't need every baby product ever marketed, there are some items that are non-negotiables. Here's a quick guide to the things you'll need in their first year.

High chair

When your baby gets older, you'll need a high chair for feeding. I've used two types of high chairs—the BudtzBendix Tower Chair (if you could call a high chair beautiful, this would be it) and the basic IKEA high chair (the one you see at every cafe, everywhere). Both are easy to wipe down, and if need be, you could even get the hose out for a high-powered clean. Look for a high chair without any fitted material or padding—you can add this later if you want, but if you get a chair with this stuff built in, it can be very tricky to clean.

Panadol and Nurofen

When your baby is a month old, medications like paracetamol and ibuprofen are safe (although you must always follow the dosage indications on the packaging). Pain relief is a must for colds, flu, teething and flying. I always have a bottle of Panadol and Nurofen handy (strawberry flavour preferably; stay away from the cherry) because you never know when you might need it. Sidenote: why don't these work as effectively on adults? One little dropper of Panadol and my babies turn from howling, feverish teethers to perfect little angels in a matter of twenty minutes. Magic.

Play mat/play gym

Little babies need somewhere to hang out, too. A soft, machine-washable play mat or play gym will stimulate their senses and give you five minutes of downtime.

Travel with a newborn

Before I had kids, I imagined that, once I had them, life would continue on pretty much as normal—just with a baby tagging along. We'd wake up in the morning, have our coffee, head to work . . . and figure out what to do with the baby somewhere along the way.

The same would go for travelling: Chris and I both loved our little getaways, so it went without saying that, once we had kids, we'd still head off to escape the Melbourne winter whenever possible. It would be easy, right? Just pop the baby in a sling, and off you go.

Ahahahahahahahaha.

Not quite.

Four kids in, I know that travelling with a newborn can be tough. It requires patience, Scout Leader packing skills and the organisational talents of top military personnel. Here's what I've learned about travelling with a newborn.

There will be baby stuff wherever you are

OK, unless you're going to the Congo (in which case: don't), you'll find everything you need for your baby at your destination. I promise.

The first time we took Oscar away, we went to Noosa. I thought I was so clever, buying a portacot and this ridiculously expensive pram suitcase to stuff our even more ridiculously expensive pram in. We had a trolley loaded with suitcases, which in turn were packed with basically everything we'd ever used with Oscar over the first few months of his life. The steriliser. Books. Toys. Enough clothes that he could have a change of outfit once every few hours, if he so desired (he did not). It was crazy.

Of course, as we manoeuvred our way around the airport, the trolley struggled to hold the weight of the bags, and eventually, they all fell off. Everyone turned to stare as Chris tried to pick them up, and I tried to soothe Oscar in the BabyBjörn (because when the shit hits the fan, it *really* hits the fan).

Chris and I almost never fight, but I swear to you: I almost called a divorce lawyer that day.

So don't pack all that useless shit. They will have nappies, formula and yes, even a cot at most destinations (though of course it's always best to check). Call ahead, hire a cot or a pram or a bouncer (or all three) and save yourself the hassle. And your marriage.

One thing you will need . . .

. . . is a comfortable baby carrier for the airport (and for settling on the plane, if necessary). I love the BabyBjörn.

Fly at night

If you're doing a long-haul flight (over eight hours), try to fly at night, when your baby will be asleep anyway. Don't worry about scoring a seat with a bassinet—most babies only fit into them when they are very, very small (my kids grew out of them at four months), and young babies fall asleep easily on you anyway (in theory—some kids seem to sense your need for them to sleep . . . and then point-blank refuse to do so).

Keep your baby on their routine

Unless you're going to the other side of the world for an extended period of time (more than a few weeks), I'd keep your baby on their current routine. This means keeping them on *their time zone*. We went to Perth with the twins when they were seven months old, and though it was torture at the start of the day (the boys woke up at 7 a.m. Melbourne time . . . which was 5 a.m. in Perth), when we got home, they went straight back into their routine without a hassle.

Before they walk or after they talk

This is the sweet spot for travelling with kids. Go before they can move (keeping a moving baby entertained on a plane = worst time ever) or after they can talk (so you can reason with them/bribe them to sit still).

What to take on the plane

* A big, purpose-made baby bag with all the bells, whistles, pockets, compartments and dooverlackies. I like the Country Road nappy bag.
* If you're formula feeding, be sure to pack lots of bottles full of sterilised, cooled water. I like to have the bottle ready to go, with the teat and lid on. If you're breastfeeding: lucky you. You've got it easy! I carry a formula dispenser with my formula measured out perfectly in each compartment. That way you just need to tip it into your pre-filled bottles, shake and warm. The flight attendants are usually pretty great at warming your bottles. Give them a heads up when you'll be requiring them to do it so it's not in the middle of a meal service and your baby is starving and screaming.
* Lots of bibs. About three more than you think is necessary.
* Puree packets, rusks and rubber spoons if your baby is on solids.
* At least two changes of clothes for baby. For some reason, babies love spewing and pooing through their clothes on long-haul flights. Just another reason to love travelling with them.
* A warm jumper and socks for baby. Planes can be so cold.
* A change of clothes for you, too. I've been caught out twice covered in spew and baby food on a plane. Never again.
* Your baby's sleeping bag or sleeping blanket. They associate these items with sleep, so they can stick to their routine, even on the plane.
* Lots of nappies and wipes.

* Hand sanitiser and antibacterial wipes to clean down the surfaces you and baby might touch.
* Panadol, Nurofen and any prescribed medication your baby needs. There is nothing worse than a screaming, sick child on a plane. I always have back-up medical supplies in case they get sick or decide to start teething when we're 30,000 feet in the air.
* Plastic bags for soiled bits and bobs.

Feed on take-off and landing

Little babies suffer the same ear blocking as we do when we're on a plane, but unlike us, they can't get rid of it on their own. The best thing to do is feed them on take-off and landing. The sucking will help them unblock their ears.

Plan for the worst

There will be delays. There will be missed connections. Even if you book a bassinet, you may not get it. Pack extra supplies and keep your expectations in check.

Be realistic

Taking little babies on long-haul flights is hard. There will be bright moments in between the craziness, but I have been known to turn to my husband when we've taken our kids overseas and tell him that we have made the absolute worst decision of our lives. Just so you know.

Go for a decent amount of time—more than ten days, I reckon. Know that things won't always go to plan, and learn to roll with that. Be patient, set your expectations a little lower than normal (cocktails at 9 p.m. and dinner at 11 are probably out of the question) and relax.

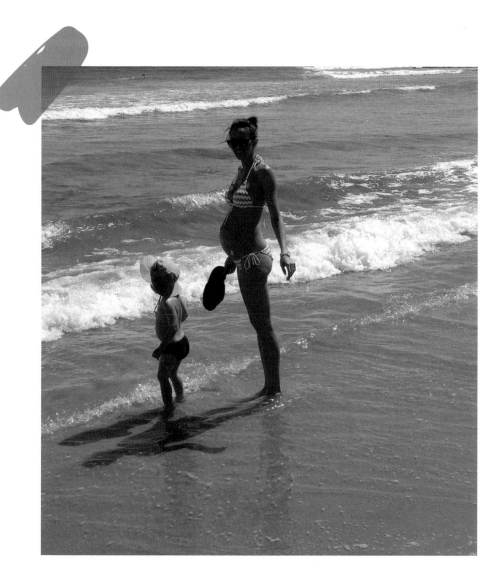

Noosa beach, with Oscar, and Billie in my belly. We didn't know it at the time but, sheesh, one kid is easy!

Mum life hacks you never knew you needed

You know those BuzzFeed articles that are like, 'Ten life hacks that will help you be a morning person'? This is the mum version of that—super helpful, totally random hints that will make your life way easier. (And guess what? You *are* a morning person now! You're a mum, you have no choice. Good hack, right?)

* Always take a book in the car. You never know when your baby will fall asleep and you'll be stuck for an hour with 4 per cent phone battery.
* Same goes for snacks and an iPhone charger (see above). I've managed to get so much work done sitting in my car in the garage because my baby is asleep.
* Kids hate sunscreen, but they love getting their faces painted. So tell your kid you're painting their face when you're applying SPF. Look, it won't work forever, but it'll get you through.
* Kids also hate getting their nails cut. My hint? Take a pair of nail clippers with you in the car—your kid will fall asleep and then you can trim their nails. (I promise, these are not all car-related.)
* As your kids get older and start reading, get the oldest one to practise their reader at story time with your younger kids. The babies get read to, the eldest does their homework (thanks, Oscar!), and you get to have a glass of wine and listen. Winning.
* When your baby starts solids, fill your freezer with huge, portioned-out batches of steamed veggies (ice-cube trays are great for portioning). Then, make up batches of pureed protein—beef mince, chicken and salmon all work well. This way, you've always got heaps of options ready to go.
* Download your favourite kids' apps (ABC 4 Kids is a goodie) and bookmark the best YouTube videos (Justine Clarke's 'Watermelon' and 'I Like to Sing' are always winners) to bring out at restaurants and cafes to keep the babies quiet.
* You know how people say, 'I've got no time to shower, with a baby'? You do. You just need to include the baby in the shower. Well, not in the shower . . . but in the bathroom. Whack your baby in a bouncer, facing you in the shower, and go for it. Cleanse, shampoo, condition—the whole nine yards. Mate, you'll even have time to exfoliate—face *and* body. Babies love

the bathroom for some reason. I would do this before my babies' first nap in the morning. Everyone had a better day once I had a wash.

* There will come a time when your baby will get fussy over food. Here's my tip: hand them a rusk (or a biscuit, or anything you know they'll open up for), and when they open their mouth to put it in, spoon the meal in, too. Works every time.

* Keep a packed nappy wallet or bag containing nappies, wipes, a bib, a spoon and a change of clothes in your pram and your car. This way, you're ready to leave at any time, and you only need to add fresh items (food or bottles if formula feeding). You'll add years to your life.

* Nappies leak . . . unless you buy them in the next size up. Do it and save yourself approximately $507 in Napisan.

* Repeat after me: white noise, white noise, white noise. Go to the App Store now, download a white noise app, and put it on when your baby goes to sleep. They work wonders.

* If you're planning on going out and leaving your baby with a carer (who doesn't have your boobies) for more than three hours—like, ever—it's good to introduce a bottle once a day in the first few weeks. Trust me, if you don't introduce the bottle early—and consistently—babies will often reject it.

* A great time to introduce the bottle is the 10 p.m. feed. A great person to do this feed is your partner. Not only will your partner get some precious bonding time with bub, you will get to go to sleep after the 6 p.m. feed . . . and sleep until the 2 a.m. feed. That's around seven hours of sleep. That's bloody brilliant.

* If your baby is sick and won't take the prescribed liquid medicine (let's face it, those oral suspension antibiotics taste like crap) check with your doctor first, and ask your pharmacist to provide the medication in a capsule form. Split the capsule open (at the required dose) and sprinkle the contents into melted ice cream, puree or milk. You'll find something that works for you.

* Swaddle your newborn baby in a muslin wrap or thin blanket and then zip them into an Ergococoon. This way they will never wriggle out of their wrap.

Final thoughts

. . . .

Oh, mama! You did it! You had a baby . . . and you made it to the end of this book. You know all about my vagina and my abs and that time I just could not hold my wee in. You took care of your baby for nine months (more like ten, really) and now that baby is here, a real little person for you to get to know and love and cherish. I like to think we've become friends. Yeah? Yeah.

While this book—and this chapter of your parenting journey—is ending, this is really just the beginning for you. Pretty soon a whole new set of challenges and obstacles will present themselves—first teeth, first days at day care, first colds (argh!) and first steps will be here before you know it. I know. All this stuff seems so far away right now, but believe me: it goes quicker than you can imagine.

So I want to end by giving you a wee bit of advice (pun intended). Enjoy it. Being a parent—and especially being a mum—can be fraught with all sorts of dangers, both real and imagined. But I really believe that the best thing you can do for your kids is to enjoy being their parent. Sometimes you won't, of course. Some days will be horrible. You'll be covered in milk spew and poo and bodily fluids you didn't even know existed. Some days your kids will drive you up the wall and you'll start asking yourself when it's appropriate to have a glass of wine at around 10 a.m.

But most days will be—when you look back on them—amazing. Your baby will soon smile, and then laugh, and then talk, and then walk. They'll start playing and listening to you as you read to them, and want to hug and kiss you goodnight. They'll run to you when they trip over and they'll fall asleep on you after a big day of playing. Enjoy it. You're a mum, and to your baby, you are among a very select group of the most special people in the world.

Of course, enjoying being a parent also means doing it your way. Some mums reading this book won't be into routines, and that is OK. Some mums won't ever want to go back to work, and that's fine, too. Some mums, like me, love the odd night out with their girlfriends, and on those nights, are happy to skip the bath-book-bed routine. Others wouldn't dream of it.

I really think that to enjoy being a parent, you have to figure out the way that suits your family best. Don't be afraid to acknowledge what this means to you, your partner and your baby.

And above all else, remember this: all your kid ever really needs is to be happy and healthy. The rest is icing on the cake. Which you should totally eat right now. And enjoy it.

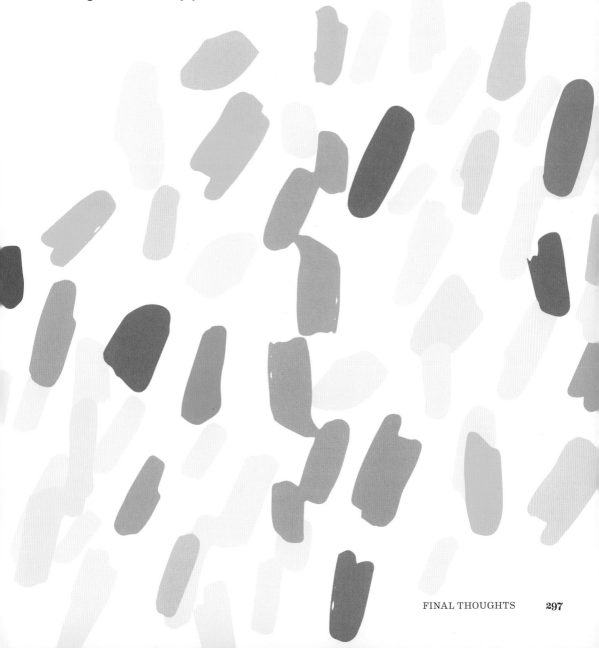

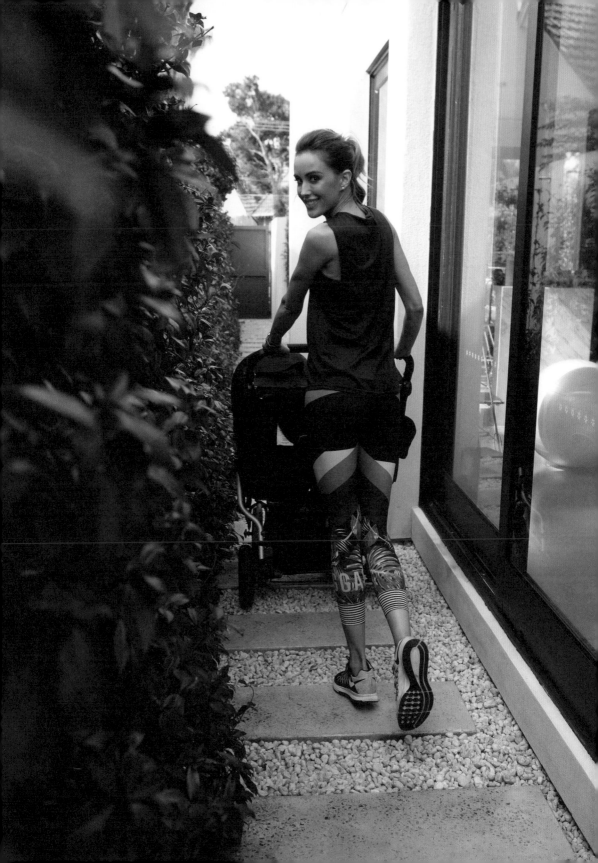

Acknowledgements

Firstly to Oscar, Billie, Tom and Darcy—the little people who made me a mum—you have all taught me so much in different ways. Just look at everything in this book; I would never have known this stuff or written this if it weren't for you. Please know that I love you all dearly and unconditionally, even when I'm yelling at you and banishing you to your rooms.

To my incredible medical and support team—Dr Len Kliman, midwife Cath Curtin, Dr Andrew Ngu, physio Shira Kramer and sleep consultant Amanda McGill—thank you for keeping me sane, healthy, strong, fit and well slept. I feel so lucky to have had the world's best in their fields in my baby team and also thank you for contributing your knowledge to my book so that other women get to share in your wisdom too.

To Lauren Sams, wordsmith extraordinaire, thank you for your ace literary skills and helping to turn my story into something funnier, more entertaining and downright page turning than I ever could have imagined. You have made this whole scary book-writing process an absolute breeze and a delight.

Thanks to my manager, Lucy Mills, for your guidance and for the gentle, prodding suggestions over the last few years to write a book. 'Nah,' I'd say. 'Not yet.' Well, the time finally came and the opportunity too when the lovely team at Allen & Unwin gave me that chance to embark on my first book and provided great vision along the way. Three cheers to team A&U!

Thanks to my girlfriend Kylie Brown for sharing your PND story with us—you are brave and inspirational. To my family and friends, thank you for still loving me even though, since having babies, I am always late, frequently cancel things at the last minute, never return phone calls and text back three weeks later. I am sorry. And lastly, to the best baby-making bloke on the planet, I love making magic with you, CJ. xxx

INDEX

A
abdominal separation *see* diastasis recti
acid reflux 60, 136
acne 47, 49, 136
air travel during pregnancy 163, 167–8
air travel with a newborn 288–92
alcohol 20, 29–30
amniocentesis 82
anaemia 32, 64
antihistamines 31
audiobooks 195
Auld, Joanne 46

B
baby bath 146
baby blues 238–9
baby brain 117
baby capsule 141, 143
baby carrier 145–6, 289
baby clothes 151, 171
baby gear 140–50, 287
baby shower 183–9
babymoon 162–8
basal body temperature (BBT) 22
Bec's recipes 123–35
Bec's workouts 98–113
bedding 156, 285
bibs 151, 172, 290
birth 198–219 *see also* labour
  breech 205, 215
  C-section *see* caesarean section
  emotions after 238–9
  not feeling connection
    to baby after 200–1, 240
  twins 202
  vacuum extraction 199, 209
  what happens after 218
  within the caul 207
birth classes 118–19
birth plan 118, 176, 178–9
blackout blinds 150
bleeding during pregnancy 52, 80, 95
bleeding gums 136
blood group and antibody screen 64
blood test 37, 64–5, 76, 80–1
  28-week 170
body mass index (BMI) 37
body temperature 33, 40
books for baby 146, 148
Borg Scale 97
bottle feeding 222, 223, 234–5, 265
  baby refusing bottle 234
  introducing bottle 235, 295
  partner doing night feed 260, 295
  topping up with 222, 234–5
  travelling 290
bottles 149
bouncer 146
Braxton Hicks contractions 136, 182, 201, 204
breast pads 175
breastfeeding 222–35
  alternate breasts 230
  baby falling asleep during 278–9
  baby refusing breast 230–1
  cluster feeding 229
  conflicting advice 236–7
  difficulties 222–4, 228, 230, 232, 234–5
  engorged breasts 222, 228–9
  expressing milk 232
  flat nipples 229
  latching 226, 232
  mastitis 71, 223, 230, 233–4
  nipple shields 229, 232–3
  positions 226
  sore breasts 222, 228–9
  tongue-tied baby 233
  topping up with formula 222, 234–5
  twins 226
breasts (during pregnancy)
  dark nipples 136
  growing 70, 71, 86, 90, 173
  leaking milk 137
  sore 23, 24, 52
Brown, Kylie 240
bunny rugs 150, 172

C
cabbage leaves for sore breasts 228, 234
caesarean section 202–4, 215–18
  birth plan 178, 179
  elective 215, 216
  emergency 216, 217
  pain relief after 218
  wound 172, 173, 203, 216
calcium 38
calories 37
car seat 141, 143
cats 32
cervical incompetence 121
cervical mucus 22
change table 143–4
  see also portable change mat
chickenpox vaccination 65
chorionic villus sampling (CVS) 82
chromosomal abnormalities, testing for 74, 80, 81
cluster feeding 229
coffee/caffeine 30

colostrum 227, 228
compression bandage 86, 90
compression shorts 173, 249
conflicting advice 236–7
constipation 57, 58, 87, 123, 136
co-sleeping 286
costs 54, 55
cot 141, 155, 284–6
crying (after birth) 238–9, 241
crying (baby) 268, 275, 280–1
Curtin, Cathryn 13, 63, 204, 222, 224, 225, 266

D
dermatitis 46
diabetes 32, 37
   gestational 32, 93, 123, 170
diarrhoea 34, 136, 165
diastasis recti 86–9, 99, 137
dietitian 36
dihydroxyacetone (DHA) 50
Down syndrome, testing for 74, 80, 81, 82
DRAM see diastasis recti
dry skin 43, 46
dummy 149, 236
Dunstan Baby Language system 281
dwarfism 177

E
eating during pregnancy 29, 34–9, 123–35
   food hygiene 35
   foods to avoid 34
   morning sickness and 58
ectopic pregnancy 80
epidural 178, 199, 200, 208–13
episiotomy 209, 216
exercise after birth 247–53
exercise during pregnancy 32–3, 40–2, 86–113
   Bec's workouts 98–113
   Borg Scale 97
   DRAM and 86–8
   exercises to avoid 95
   first trimester 40
   pelvic floor 15, 40–2, 96, 99
   safe exercise 93
   second trimester 90–2
   third trimester 169
   twin pregnancy 91, 92
expressing milk 232

F
facial hair 136
feeding pillow 145
feeding pyjamas 175
feeding tops 175
ferritin levels 65
fibre 57, 123, 176
finding out baby's sex 75–8, 84, 121

first antenatal visit 64–5
foetal abnormalities 121, 177
foetal alcohol syndrome 30
folate 38
food see eating during pregnancy
formula feeding 222, 223, 234–5
full blood examination 64

G
genetic study 121
genetic testing 74, 81
gestational diabetes 32, 93, 123, 170
getting pregnant 20, 22, 24

H
haemorrhoids 57–8
hair dyes 49–50
hepatitis test 65
high chair 287
high-waisted knickers 172, 249
HIV test 65
home birth 54
hospital see also birth; labour
   admission to 207
   birth centres 55
   costs 55
   going home from 218
   packing bag for 171–6
   private room 54
   taking baby home from 254
   visitors at 237
   when to go to 205–6, 207
human chorionic gonadotropin (hCG) 26
hydrocephalus 177
hydronephrosis 177
hydroquinone 47

I
incontinence 41, 89, 136
indigestion 160
induction 199–200
insect repellent 168
iodine 39
iron 37, 38, 65
itchy skin 43

J
jet lag 63

K
kidney disease, testing for 65
Kligman's formula 47
Kliman, Dr Len 12, 29, 36, 40, 49, 54, 57, 61, 64, 74, 199, 200, 201
Kramer, Shira 15, 41, 86, 87, 93, 248, 249

L
labour 198–219
   coaching through pushing 214
   dilation of cervix 199, 200, 204, 208

labour continued

early 201, 204–5
epidural 178, 199, 200, 208–13
feeling of contractions 189, 199, 208–9
induced 199–200
length of 214
monitoring baby during 214
not recognising signs of 201
pain relief 118, 178, 200, 208–9
pooing during 214
prenatal classes about 118
pushing during 212, 213, 214
sex causing premature 30
signs of 204–5
treatment of midwife 215
waters breaking 198, 205, 206
waters not breaking 206
when to go to hospital 205–6
lactation 227
laser treatments 44, 48, 59
laxatives 57
Leader, Tahna 268
listeria 34, 35

M

McGill, Amanda 16, 268, 269
massages 44–4, 163
mastitis 71, 223, 230, 233–4
maternity bras 72, 173, 228
maternity clothes 70–2
maternity pads 175, 249
Maxolon 58
medicine, getting baby to take 295
melasma 46, 47–8
mid-stream urine test 65
Midwife Cath see Curtin, Cathryn
morning sickness 57, 58–9, 63, 84
Moro reflex 266, 267, 280
multiples see twins
multivitamins 37–8
mum life hacks 294–5
muslin wraps 150, 172
myths about pregnancy 78

N

nail cutting 254, 284
nappies 144, 171, 295
nappy bags 145, 149
nappy rash cream 144
nausea 52, 58–9, 63
Ngu, Dr Andrew 14, 66, 67, 79, 120, 177
nipple shields 229, 232–3
non-invasive prenatal test (NIPT) 76, 81
nosebleeds 23, 28, 136
Nurofen 31, 287, 291
nursery 152–9

nursing bras 72, 173, 228
nursing chair 145, 154

O

oestrogen 59
onesies 151, 171
ovulation 22, 24

P

packing hospital bag 171–6
pain in pelvis 80
pain relief after birth 218, 228
pain relief during labour 118, 178, 208–13
pain relief during pregnancy 31
pain relief for baby 287, 291
Panadol 31, 287, 291
pap smears 56
pelvic floor 15, 28, 40, 41, 88, 89, 248
exercises 40–2, 96, 99, 250
pigmentation changes 46, 47
Pilates 40, 63, 86, 90, 91, 94, 96, 251
placenta delivery 179, 227
placenta failing 200
placenta position 120
placenta previa 33
play mat/play gym 287
portable change mat 146
post-birth body 91, 244, 246–7
postnatal depression 239–43
pram 140–1
pre-eclampsia 32, 215, 217
pregnancy hormones 26, 41, 46, 116
pregnancy mask 47
pregnancy massage 44–5, 163
pregnancy symptoms 23, 28, 52, 57–60, 136–7
prenatal classes 118–19
private health insurance 55
progesterone 46, 60, 123
public or private patient 54–6
pyridoxine 58

R

reading to baby 146, 148, 294
recipes 126–35
recovery after birth 244–53
reflux (baby) 223, 256, 281
reflux during pregnancy 60, 136, 160
retinoid/retinol 47, 49, 59
RICER principle 249
rosacea 46, 48
routines 256–65, 268–74
'feed-play-sleep' 261, 270, 274, 276, 278
impediments 273–4
newborn 261–2, 269–74
travel and 289
twins 264–5, 268
when to start 258, 269

rubella antibody status 64
ruptured membranes 33

S

salicylic acids 49
setting up home for baby 194–5
sex during pregnancy 30–1, 84, 97, 137
shared care 54
showering with baby 294–5
SIDS/SUDI 283–6
skincare during pregnancy 43–51
sleep (baby) 256–86
  awake time 257, 278
  circadian rhythm 269, 275
  co-sleeping 286
  crying 268, 275, 280–1
  cues 257, 258–9
  cycles 279
  falling asleep while feeding 278
  feeding to sleep 275, 276
  independent sleep skills 276
  newborn routine 261–2, 269–74
  overtiredness 258
  patterns 279
  poor sleeping habits 275
  professional help 256, 263, 268, 282
  routines 257–65, 268–74
  safe sleeping tips 283–6
  self-settling 268, 275, 280
  sharing a room 286
  sleeping position 285
  swaddling 260, 266–7, 280, 285, 295
  unsettledness 280–1
  white noise 279, 295
sleep consultant 256, 263, 268, 282
sleeping bag 150, 285
spa baths 33
spider veins 137
spina bifida 33
steriliser 148
stitches after birth 216
Stratamark cream 44
stretch marks 44, 46, 47, 59
sucking blister 225
sucking reflex 180, 225, 266, 280
Sudocrem 144
sunscreen 47, 48, 294
swaddles 150
swaddling 260, 266–7, 280, 285, 295
sudden infant death syndrome (SIDS) 283–6
sudden unexplained death in infancy (SUDI) 283–6
syphilis serology 65

T

tests during pregnancy 64–5, 74, 76, 80–2, 170
thalassemia 64

thermometer 150
thyroid function 37, 39, 65
tiredness 28, 52, 114
tongue-tie 233
toxoplasmosis 32
travel cot 148, 288
travel during pregnancy 162–8
travel with newborn 288–93
tretinoin 47
trisomy conditions 74
TSH levels 65
twins 61–3, 66–7
  breastfeeding 226
  exercise during pregnancy 91, 92
  giving birth to 182, 202
  identical/non-identical 66, 67
  monochorionic diamniotic (MCDA) 67
  monochorionic monoamniotic (MCMA) 67
  risks 66
  routine 264–5, 268
  sleeping arrangements 286
  twin-to-twin transfusion syndrome (TTTS) 82–3
  ultrasounds 82–3

U

ultrasounds 79–83, 120–2, 177
  finding out baby's sex 75, 76, 84, 121
  first trimester 79–83
  second trimester 120–2
  third trimester 177

V

vacuum extraction 199, 209
vaginal discharge 136, 172, 205
vaginal tear 209
varicella serology 65
varicose veins 57, 60, 137
visitors 237
vitamins 29, 38, 58
  vitamin A 43, 49
  vitamin B 38, 48, 58
  vitamin D 37, 38, 65
  vitamin K shot (for baby) 218
vulvar varices 60

W

water retention 160
waters breaking 198, 205, 206
waters not breaking 206
wetting your pants 136, 165, 182
white noise 279, 295
wipes 140, 144, 146, 171, 295
wrapping baby 266–7, 280, 285, 295

Y

Yates, Suzanne 45

Z

Zofran 58

First published in 2018

Allen & Unwin
83 Alexander Street
Crows Nest NSW 2065
Australia
Phone: (61 2) 8425 0100
Email: info@allenandunwin.com
Web: www.allenandunwin.com

A catalogue record for this book is available from the National Library of Australia

NATIONAL LIBRARY OF AUSTRALIA

ISBN 978 1 76063 130 7

Internal design and illustration by Miriam Steenhauer
Food styling by Deborah Kaloper
All photos are courtesy of Bec Judd unless otherwise indicated.
pp. 4, 186, 187 (Liane Hurvitz); pp. 6, 142, 154, 155, 157, 159 (Julie Adams); p. 35 (Pixabay); pp. 42, 45, 98, 101, 105, 106, 108, 111, 125, 127, 128, 131, 132, 135, 252, 298 (Ed Purnomo); p. 59 (iStock); p. 124 (Stocksy); pp. 184, 189 (Lauren Crouch)
Backgrounds by Shutterstock and iStock
Index by Puddingburn
Printed by C&C Offset Printing Co. Ltd, China

10 9 8 7 6 5 4 3 2

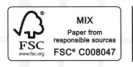